CW00515044

© Copyright 2020 by ANNIE kELLER - All rights reserved.

The following Book is reproduced below with the goal of providing information that is as accurate and reliable as possible. Regardless, purchasing this Book can be seen as consent to the fact that both the publisher and the author of this book are in no way experts on the topics discussed within and that any recommendations or suggestions that are made herein are for entertainment purposes only. Professionals should be consulted as needed prior to undertaking any of the action endorsed herein.

This declaration is deemed fair and valid by both the American Bar Association and the Committee of Publishers Association and is legally binding throughout the United States.

Furthermore, the transmission, duplication, or reproduction of any of the following work including specific information will be considered an illegal act irrespective of if it is done electronically or in print. This extends to creating a secondary or tertiary copy of the work or a recorded copy and is only allowed with the express written consent from the Publisher. All additional right reserved.

The information in the following pages is broadly considered a truthful and accurate account of facts and as such, any inattention, use, or misuse of the information in question by the reader will render any resulting actions solely under their purview. There are no scenarios in which the publisher or the original author of this work can be in any fashion deemed liable for any hardship or damages that may befall them after undertaking information described herein.

Additionally, the information in the following pages is intended only for informational purposes and should thus be thought of as universal. As befitting its nature, it is presented without assurance regarding its prolonged validity or interim quality. Trademarks that are mentioned are done without written consent and can in no way be considered an endorsement from the trademark holder.

VEGAN COOKING:

50 Recipes to Get You Started!

ANNIE KELLER

Table of Contents

THE FAVORITES - VEGAN STYLE
Cheese-Stuffed Meatballs
Ultimate Twice-Baked Potatoes
Double-Double Cheeseburgers

BALANCED VEGAN
Chinese Chickpea Salad
Pecan Pesto Spaghetti Squash with Peas & Kale
Chile-Roasted Tofu Lettuce Cups
Buddha Bowl

HOMESTYLE VEGAN
Chickpea & Dumplin' Soup
Shiitake Stroganoff
Unstuffed Cabbage Rolls

VEGAN CLASSICS
Balsamic-Roasted Beet & Cheese Galette
French Onion Soup
Truffled Mashed Potato–Stuffed Portobellos

VEGAN SANDWICHES
Fillet o' Chickpea Sandwich with Tartar Sauce Slaw
The Portobello Philly Reuben
BBQ Pulled Jackfruit Sandwich

VEGAN BAKING
Blueberry-Banana Muffins
Chocolate Layer Cake
Peanut Butter Oatmeal Cookies

VEGAN COMFORT FOOD
Hash Brown Casserole (aka Company Potatoes)

Roasted Carrot & Wild Mushroom Ragout
Sweet Potato Shepherd's Pie

VEGAN FOR PICKY EATERS
Artichoke-Kale Hummus
BLT Summer Rolls with Avocado
Perfect Roasted Potatoes

GAME DAY VEGAN
Buffalo Cauliflower Wings with Blue Cheese Dip
Jalapeño Popper Bites
Cheesy Spiced Popcorn
Chickpea-Avocado Taquitos

GET-TOGETHER VEGAN MEALS
Avocado & Hearts of Palm Tea Sandwiches
Roasted Red Pepper Hummus Cucumber Cups
Chickpea Caesar Pasta Salad
Sun-Dried Tomato & White Bean Bruschetta

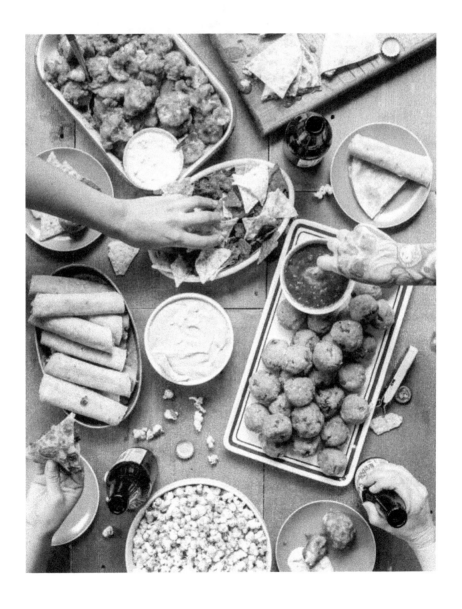

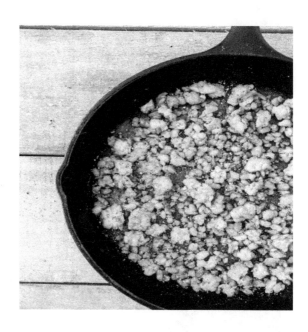

Quick Bacon Crumbles

MAKES 2 CUPS

PREP TIME: **5 minutes**
ACTIVE TIME: **30 minutes**

One 8-oz. Package tempeh (soy-free if necessary)
¼ cup liquid aminos (or gluten-free tamari; use coconut
aminos to be soy-free)
¼ cup low-sodium vegetable broth
2 tablespoons olive oil
1 tablespoon liquid smoke
1 tablespoon maple syrup
½ teaspoon ground cumin
½ teaspoon garlic powder
Black pepper to taste

1. Line a plate with paper towels. Crumble the tempeh into
small pieces and set aside.

2. Combine the liquid aminos, broth, 1 tablespoon of the olive oil, the liquid smoke, maple syrup, cumin, and garlic powder in a cup. Stir until combined.

3. Heat the remaining olive oil in a large frying pan, preferably cast iron, over medium heat. Add the tempeh crumbles and toss to coat in oil. Cook for about 1 minute, then add the sauce. Cook, stirring every few minutes, until the liquid has been absorbed and the tempeh is tender with a crispy exterior.

4. Transfer the tempeh to the prepared plate to absorb any excess oil. Sprinkle with black pepper. Serve immediately. Leftovers will keep in an airtight container in the fridge for 4 to 5 days.

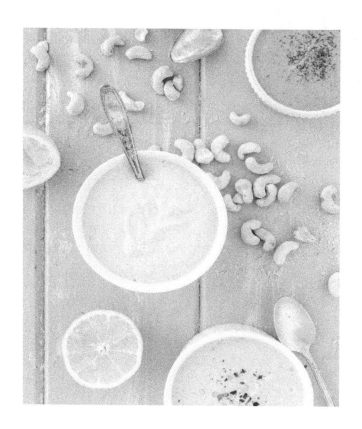

Basic Cashew Cheese Sauce

MAKES ¾ CUP

PREP TIME: **5 minutes**
ACTIVE TIME: **10 minutes**
INACTIVE TIME: **60 minutes**

½ cup raw cashews, soaked in warm water for at least 1 hour and drained, water reserved

5 to 6 tablespoons reserved soaking water

2 tablespoons lemon juice

2 tablespoons nutritional yeast

½ teaspoon white soy miso (or chickpea miso)

Combine the cashews, ¼ cup of the reserved soaking water, the lemon juice, nutritional yeast, and miso in a food processor or blender and process until smooth. Add up to 2 tablespoons more water for a thinner sauce. Store in an airtight container in the refrigerator for up to 7 days. The cheese will thicken when chilled, so you may need to add more water to thin it back out (unless you want a cheese spread, as described in the Variations).

VARIATIONS

Smoked Gouda Cheese Sauce: Add 1 teaspoon smoked paprika, ½ teaspoon garlic powder, and ½ teaspoon dried dill.

Pepperjack Cheese Sauce: Add ½ teaspoon onion powder, ½ teaspoon garlic powder, and 1 teaspoon red pepper flakes.

Mixed Herb Cheese Sauce: Add 2 teaspoons dried mixed herbs of your choice. I prefer ½ teaspoon dried thyme, ½ teaspoon dried parsley, ½ teaspoon dried oregano, and ½ teaspoon dried basil, but any blend will do.

Melty Cheese: For cheese that seems melty and browns when baked—for the main recipe or any of the variations—increase the water to ⅔ cup and add 1 tablespoon arrowroot powder or cornstarch. Transfer the cheese to a small pot and heat over medium heat, stirring constantly, 3 to 4 minutes, until it's thickened but still drips slowly off a spoon. Pour it on top of whatever you're baking and proceed with that recipe's instructions.

Cheese Spread: Use only 3 tablespoons water, or use the regular amount and chill the cheese sauce for at least 24 hours. The sauce will thicken into a spread.

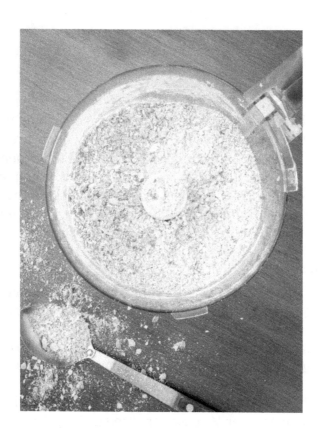

Pepita Parmesan

MAKES 3 CUPS

PREP TIME: 5 minutes
ACTIVE TIME: **2 minutes**

2½ cups pepitas (pumpkin seeds)
½ cup nutritional yeast
1½ teaspoons lemon juice

Combine all of the ingredients in a food processor and pulse until broken down into a coarse powder. Transfer to an airtight container. Leftovers will keep in the fridge for up to 2 weeks.

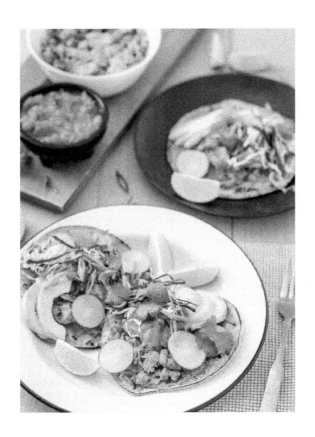

Tofu Rancheros

SERVES 4 OR 5

PREP TIME: 10 minutes (not including time to make 15-Minute
Refried   Beans)
  ACTIVE TIME: 20 minutes

1 teaspoon olive oil
½ medium yellow onion, diced
One 14-ounce block extra firm tofu
2 tablespoons vegetable broth, plus more if needed
1 teaspoon black salt (kala namak; or regular salt)
1 teaspoon ground cumin
½ teaspoon paprika
¼ teaspoon ground turmeric
3 tablespoons nutritional yeast, optional
1 tablespoon lemon juice
Black pepper to taste

rancheros

8 to 10 corn tortillas (2 per person)

½ batch _15-Minute Refried Beans_

Salsa
Chopped fresh cilantro
Sliced avocado, optional
Shredded cabbage or lettuce, optional
Sliced radishes, optional
Chopped green onions, optional
Lime wedges

1. **To make the scrambled tofu:** Heat the olive oil in a large skillet over medium heat. Add the onion and sauté for 3-4 minutes. Crumble the tofu into the pan. Cook, stirring gently, until the tofu is no longer releasing any water and is starting to brown on the edges, about 10 minutes. Meanwhile, combine broth, black salt, cumin, paprika, and turmeric in a small cup.

2. Once the tofu has stopped releasing water, add the broth mixture. Cook for about 5 minutes more, until the liquid is absorbed. If it begins to stick, add another tablespoon of broth to deglaze the pan and reduce the heat. Add the nutritional yeast (if using) and lemon juice and cook for about 1 minute more. Remove from the heat and cover the pan to keep warm.

3. **To make the rancheros:** Heat a small pan over medium heat. Place a tortilla in the pan and cook for about 1 minute, flip it, and cook for about 30 seconds more. Transfer to a plate and cover with aluminum foil. Repeat with the remaining tortillas.

4. Spread some refried beans over each tortilla. Top with tofu scramble, a little salsa, and cilantro. If desired, you can also top with avocado slices, shredded cabbage, radish slices, and/or green onions. Serve immediately with a lime wedge. Any leftover scramble can be kept in an airtight container in the fridge for 3 to 4 days.

Maple–Peanut Butter Pancakes

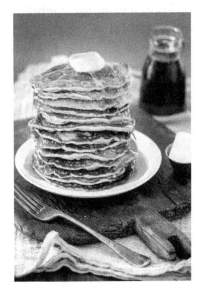

MAKES 8 PANCAKES

PREP TIME: **10 minutes**
ACTIVE TIME: **25 minutes**

¾ cup oat flour (certified gluten-free)
¾ cup gluten-free flour blend (soy-free if necessary)
1 tablespoon cornstarch
1 tablespoon baking powder
½ teaspoon salt
1¼ cups nondairy milk (nut-free and/or soy-free if necessary)
1⅓ cup maple syrup, plus more for serving

¼ cup unsalted, unsweetened peanut butter (or nut or seed butter of your choice)
1 tablespoon apple cider vinegar
1 teaspoon vanilla extract
Vegan cooking spray (soy-free if necessary)
Vegan butter (soy-free if necessary), optional

1. If you're not serving the pancakes immediately, see Tip below. In a large bowl, whisk together the oat flour, gluten-free flour, cornstarch, baking powder, and salt. In a medium bowl, whisk together the milk, maple syrup, peanut butter, vinegar, and vanilla. Add the wet ingredients to the dry and stir until combined.

2. Heat a large frying pan or griddle over medium heat for a couple of minutes. Lightly spray with cooking spray. Using a ⅓-cup measuring cup, scoop the batter onto the pan and cook until the top begins to bubble and the edges begin to lift. Use a spatula to flip the pancake. Cook for another minute or two. Gently lift the edge of the pancake to make sure it's golden brown, then transfer the pancake to a plate (or the oven, as in Tip below). Repeat with the remaining batter, taking care to regrease the pan between pancakes.

3. Serve the pancakes topped with a bit of butter (if desired) and a drizzle of maple syrup. Keep leftovers in an airtight container in the fridge for 1 to 2 days.

VARIATIONS

▶ These can also be made by replacing the oat flour, gluten-free flour, and cornstarch with 1½ cups unbleached all-purpose flour. If the batter is too thick, you may need to add a few tablespoons of nondairy milk to thin it out.

▶ You can also use this batter to make waffles by cooking it in a waffle maker according to the machine instructions.

If you're not planning to serve the pancakes right away, preheat the oven to its lowest setting before you start preparing your batter. Place a cooling rack on a baking sheet. Once a pancake is done, transfer it to the cooling rack and place the sheet in the oven. Continue transferring all pancakes to the rack (avoiding overlapping if possible) and keep them there for up to 20 minutes.

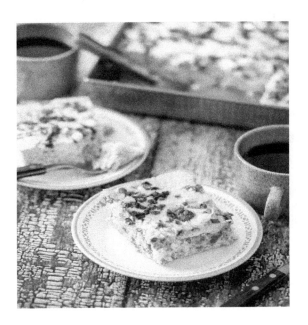

Savory Breakfast Casserole

SERVES 10 TO 12

PREP TIME: **10 minutes** (not including time to make Quick Bacon Crumbles)
ACTIVE TIME: **20 minutes**
INACTIVE TIME: **40 to 45 minutes**

Olive oil spray

One 14-ounce block extra firm tofu
3 cups unsweetened nondairy milk (nut-free if necessary)
2½ cups chickpea flour
2 tablespoons lemon juice
2 tablespoons nutritional yeast
1½ teaspoons black salt (kala namak; or regular salt)
1½ teaspoons garlic powder
1 teaspoon mustard powder
¾ teaspoon ground turmeric
Black pepper to taste
1 teaspoon olive oil
½ medium yellow onion, diced
1 red bell pepper, diced
One 16-ounce bag frozen hash browns
Quick Bacon Crumbles

4 green onions, chopped (green and white parts)

1. Preheat the oven to 400°F. Lightly spray a 9 × 13-inch baking dish with olive oil.

2. Gently squeeze the tofu over the sink, releasing any extra water. Add the tofu, milk, chickpea flour, lemon juice, nutritional yeast, salt, garlic powder, mustard powder, turmeric, and pepper to a blender and blend until smooth. Pour into your largest bowl.

3. Heat the olive oil in a large frying pan over medium heat. Add the onion and bell pepper and sauté until just barely tender. Pour them into the bowl and return the pan to the stove. Add the hash browns to the pan and cook for about 5 minutes, stirring occasionally, until thawed and golden in color. Remove from the heat and pour into the bowl.

4. Add the bacon crumbles to the bowl and stir until combined. Pour into the prepared baking dish and sprinkle the green onions over the top. Bake for 35 minutes, or until firm and a toothpick inserted in the center comes out clean. Remove from the oven and let rest for 5 to 10 minutes before serving. Leftovers will keep in an airtight container in the fridge for 4 to 5 days.

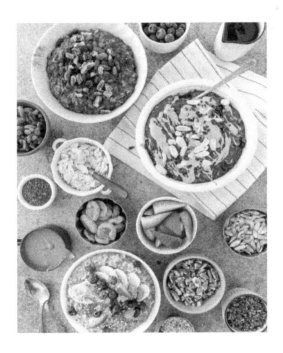

Everyone's Favorite Oatmeal

SERVES 1

PREP TIME: **2 minutes**
ACTIVE TIME: **8 minutes**

1½ cups water

1 cup rolled oats (certified gluten-free if necessary; see Tip)
¼ cup nondairy milk (nut-free and/or soy-free if necessary)
1 to 2 tablespoons maple syrup
1 teaspoon ground cinnamon
Salt to taste

1. Combine the water and oats in a small saucepan or pot and bring to a boil. Reduce to a simmer and cook, untouched, for 3 to 4 minutes, until slightly thick and sticky.

2. Add the milk, maple syrup, cinnamon, and salt and cook for 1 to 2 minutes more, until it's heated through and has reached your desired thickness. Remove from the heat and transfer to a serving bowl. Serve immediately with your choice of toppings.

VARIATIONS

Simple Fruit and Nut Oatmeal: Once cooked, top oatmeal with ⅓ cup fresh fruit (sliced banana, chopped strawberries, sliced nectarine or peach, blueberries, raspberries, blackberries) and/or 2 tablespoons chopped dried fruit (peaches, apricots, apple, cherries, raisins) and/or 1 tablespoon chopped nuts (almonds, pecans, walnuts, cashews, peanuts, macadamia nuts). If desired, drizzle with a little more maple syrup.

Cinnamon Raisin Oatmeal: Increase the amount of cinnamon to 1½ teaspoons and add 1 tablespoon blackstrap molasses and ¼ cup raisins to the oatmeal when you add the milk. Top with an additional 1 tablespoon raisins, a drizzle of maple syrup, and/or 1 tablespoon chopped nuts.

Peanut Butter and Banana Oatmeal: When adding the milk, add ⅓ cup sliced bananas and 1 tablespoon peanut butter. Top with a few more banana slices, 1 tablespoon chopped peanuts, and drizzles of peanut butter and maple syrup. You could also add a couple of tablespoons of chocolate chips to take it over the top.

▶ Double Chocolate Oatmeal: Stir in 2 tablespoons cocoa powder when you add the milk. After removing from the heat, stir in 1 to 2 tablespoons chocolate chips. Top with chopped nuts and/or cacao nibs.

▶ Fruit Pie Oatmeal: Add ⅓ cup chopped fruit of your choice (apple, pear, strawberries, bananas, blueberries, blackberries, cherries, peach, pear, persimmon) to the pot when adding the oats. Top with ¼ cup of the same fruit and/or 1 tablespoon chopped nuts.

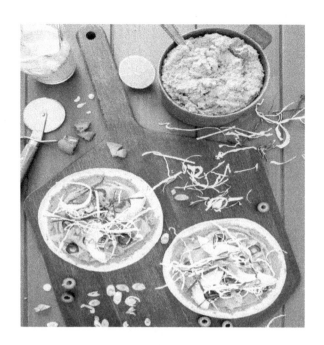

Mexican Pizza with 15-Minute Refried Beans

MAKES 4 PIZZAS, WITH EXTRA BEANS

PREP TIME: **15** (not including time to make Pepperjack Cheese Sauce)
ACTIVE TIME: **25**

15-minute refried beans
1 teaspoon olive oil
1 medium yellow onion, chopped
3 15-ounce cans pinto beans, rinsed and drained
2 tablespoons liquid aminos (or gluten-free tamari; use coconut aminos to be soy-free)
2 teaspoons ground cumin

2 teaspoons ancho chile powder

1½ teaspoons ground coriander

¾ teaspoon smoked paprika

½ cup low-sodium vegetable broth

3 tablespoons canned diced green chiles

2 tablespoons lime juice

Salt and black pepper to taste

pizzas

4 flour tortillas (rice flour or corn tortillas to make them gluten-free; if using corn tortillas, use 2 per person)

Pepperjack Cheese Sauce

1 cup chopped fresh tomatoes

½ cup sliced pitted black olives, optional

Optional toppings: sliced avocado, chopped or shredded greens of your choice, chopped green onions, Pickled Red Cabbage & Onion Relish

1. Preheat the oven to 400°F. Line one or two baking sheets with aluminum foil or silicone baking mats. Set aside.

2. **To make the refried beans:** Heat the olive oil in a large shallow saucepan over medium heat. Add the onion and sauté until just translucent, 3 to 4 minutes. Add the beans, liquid aminos, cumin, chile powder, coriander, paprika, and broth. Cook for about 5 minutes, until heated through and about half of the liquid has been absorbed.

3. Add the green chiles and lime juice and remove from the heat. Transfer to a food processor and pulse until the beans are mostly smooth with some chunks. Add salt and pepper.

4. **To make the pizzas:** Spread out the tortillas on the baking sheets. Spread refried beans generously over each one. Drizzle the cheese sauce over the beans and sprinkle the chopped tomatoes and olives (if using) over each pizza. Bake for 10 minutes, or until the tortillas are crispy.

5. Top the pizzas with your additional toppings and serve immediately. Leftover beans can be kept in an airtight container in the fridge for 5 to 6 days or frozen for up to 2 months. When reheating, you may need to add a few tablespoons of broth or water to thin them out again.

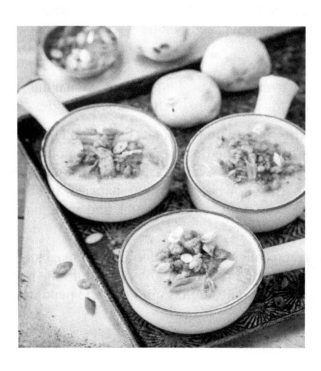

Potato Leek Soup

SERVES 4 TO 6

PREP TIME: **15 minutes** (not including time to make Quick Bacon Crumbles)
ACTIVE TIME: **25 minutes**
INACTIVE TIME: **15 minutes**

1 teaspoon olive oil
2 leeks, thinly sliced (white and light green parts)
1 garlic clove, minced
2 pounds Yukon gold potatoes, chopped
2 teaspoons dried rosemary
2 teaspoons dried thyme
1 teaspoon ground sage
3 cups low-sodium vegetable broth
2 cups water
1 tablespoon nutritional yeast, optional
1 tablespoon lemon juice
1 teaspoon liquid smoke
Salt and black pepper to taste
Quick Bacon Crumbles, optional
Chopped green onions, optional

1. In a large pot, heat the olive oil over medium heat. Add the leeks and sauté until soft, about 4 minutes. Add the garlic and sauté for another minute. Add the potatoes, rosemary, thyme, sage, broth, and water. Bring to a boil, then reduce the heat and simmer until the potatoes are tender, about 15 minutes. Turn off the heat.

2. Add the nutritional yeast, lemon juice, and liquid smoke. Use an immersion blender to blend the soup until smooth (or mostly smooth with a few potato chunks—your call). Alternatively, you can transfer the soup in batches to a blender and carefully blend until smooth.

3. Add salt and pepper. Serve topped with bacon crumbles and green onions, if desired. Leftovers will keep in an airtight container in the fridge for 5 to 6 days.

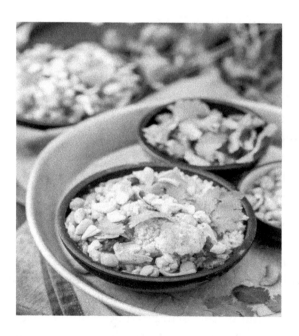

Quick Cauliflower Curry

SERVES 4 TO 6

PREP TIME: **20 minutes**
ACTIVE TIME: **15 minutes**
INACTIVE TIME: **10 minutes**

1 tablespoon coconut oil
1 medium yellow onion, diced
2 garlic cloves, minced
1 tablespoon grated fresh ginger
1 tablespoon curry powder
2 teaspoons garam masala
1 teaspoon ground coriander
1 teaspoon ground cumin
½ teaspoon ground turmeric
1 medium (1-pound head cauliflower, broken into florets
8 ounces cremini mushrooms (or button mushrooms), sliced
One 15-ounce can chickpeas, rinsed and drained
One 15-ounce can no-salt-added fire-roasted diced tomatoes
3 cups low-sodium vegetable broth
1 cup plain coconut yogurt (preferably unsweetened)
Salt and black pepper to taste
Chopped fresh cilantro, optional
Chopped cashews, optional (see Variation)
Cooked rice (or vegan bread)

1. Heat the coconut oil in a large pot or Dutch oven over medium heat. Add the onion, garlic, and ginger and sauté until the onion is just becoming translucent. Add the curry powder, garam masala, coriander, cumin, and turmeric and cook until fragrant, about 1 minute.

2. Add the cauliflower, mushrooms, chickpeas, tomatoes and their liquid, and the broth and bring to a boil. Reduce the heat to a simmer and cover. Cook for about 10 minutes, then remove the lid and cook for about 5 minutes more. Stir in the yogurt and cook for a few minutes, until heated through. Add salt and pepper and remove from the heat.

3. Top with chopped cilantro and/or cashews, if desired, and serve with rice or bread. Store leftovers in an airtight container in the fridge for 4 to 5 days.

VARIATION

To make this nut-free, switch out the cashews with pepitas (pumpkin seeds) or sesame seeds.

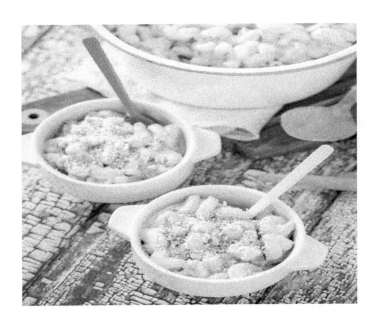

Hidden Veggie Mac 'n' Cheese

SERVES 8

PREP TIME: **15 minutes** (not including time make Pepita Parmesan)
ACTIVE TIME: **30 minutes**

½ medium (1-pound) head cauliflower, broken into florets
2 large carrots, peeled and chopped
½ cup diced radishes
1 pound elbow macaroni (gluten-free if necessary)
1 cup cooked great Northern beans
1 cup unsweetened nondairy milk (nut-free and/or soy-free if necessary)
¾ cup nutritional yeast
¼ cup lemon juice
2 tablespoons no-salt-added tomato paste

2 tablespoons vegan butter (soy-free if necessary), melted
2 teaspoons white soy miso (or chickpea miso)
1 teaspoon onion powder
1 teaspoon garlic powder
½ teaspoon paprika
¼ teaspoon mustard powder
Salt and black pepper to taste
Pepita Parmesan, optional

1. Place the cauliflower, carrots, and radishes in a medium pot and cover with water. Bring to a boil and cook the vegetables until easily pierced with a fork, 8 to 10 minutes. Remove from the heat and drain. Set aside.

2. Fill a large pot with water and bring to a boil. Once boiling, add the pasta and cook according to the package instructions until al dente. Remove from the heat, drain well, and return the pasta to the pot.

3. Transfer the vegetables to a food processor or blender. Add the beans, milk, nutritional yeast, lemon juice, tomato paste, butter, miso, onion powder, garlic powder, paprika, and mustard powder. Process until smooth. Add the sauce to the cooked pasta and stir to combine. Return to the stove and heat over medium heat, stirring occasionally, for 3 to 4 minutes, until heated through and the sauce has thickened. Serve immediately topped with Pepita Parmesan (if using). Refrigerate any leftovers in an airtight container for 4 to 5 days.

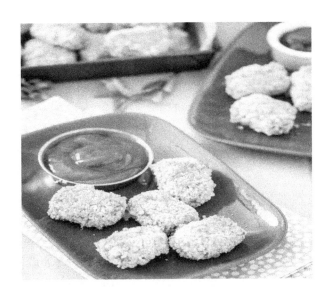

Tempeh Nuggets

MAKES 40 NUGGETS

PREP TIME: **10 minutes**
ACTIVE TIME: **30 minutes**
INACTIVE TIME: **30 minutes**

Two 8-ounce packages tempeh
3 cups low-sodium "no-chicken" flavored vegetable broth (or regular vegetable broth)
2 tablespoons liquid aminos
1 teaspoon dried thyme
1 teaspoon dried marjoram
¾ cup plain vegan yogurt (preferably unsweetened, nut-free if necessary)
¼ cup unsweetened nondairy milk (nut-free if necessary)
3 tablespoons tahini (gluten-free if necessary)
½ teaspoon salt
½ teaspoon onion powder

½ teaspoon garlic powder

¼ teaspoon smoked paprika

1½ cups vegan panko bread crumbs (gluten-free if necessary)

3 tablespoons nutritional yeast

Olive oil spray

Ketchup (or vegan barbecue sauce; homemade or store-bought), for dipping

1. Chop each block of tempeh into about 20 chunks, making 40 total nuggets.

2. Combine the broth, liquid aminos, thyme, and marjoram in a large pot. Place the tempeh in the pot and bring to a boil. Once boiling, reduce to a simmer and let the tempeh simmer for about 20 minutes. Remove from the heat and drain (you can save the liquid for another time you need to cook with broth or add a bit of liquid to your pan; it should keep in the fridge for a couple of weeks). Set the tempeh aside to cool until you can handle it.

3. While the tempeh is cooling, combine the yogurt, milk, tahini, salt, onion powder, garlic powder, and paprika in a shallow bowl. In another shallow bowl, combine the bread crumbs and nutritional yeast.

4. Preheat the oven to 375°F. Line a baking sheet with parchment paper or a silicone baking mat.

5. Use one hand to dredge a piece of tempeh in the yogurt mixture and your other hand to toss it in the bread crumbs until fully coated. Place the nugget on the prepared baking sheet. Repeat with the remaining nuggets.

6. Lightly spray the tops of the nuggets with olive oil. Bake for 12 minutes, flip them and spray the tops with olive oil again, and return to the oven for 12 minutes more, or until crispy and golden. Serve immediately with your choice of dipping sauces. Leftovers will keep in an airtight container in the fridge for 3 to 4 days.

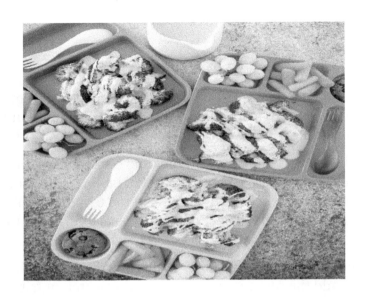

Cheesy Trees

SERVES 4, WITH EXTRA SAUCE

PREP TIME: **10 minutes**
ACTIVE TIME: **15 minutes**
INACTIVE TIME: **60 minutes**

1 cup chopped Yukon gold potatoes
½ cup peeled, chopped carrot
1 bunch (1 pound) broccoli chopped into florets
¼ cup raw cashews, soaked in warm water for 1 hour and drained, water reserved
¾ cup reserved soaking water
¼ cup nutritional yeast
2 tablespoons lemon juice
1 tablespoon olive oil
½ teaspoon onion powder

½ teaspoon garlic powder

½ teaspoon salt

Salt and black pepper to taste

1. Place the potatoes and carrots in a medium pot and cover with water. Bring to a boil and cook for 8 to 10 minutes, until the vegetables are easily pierced with a fork.

2. While you're boiling the potatoes and carrots, place the broccoli in a steamer basket over a pot of boiling water and cover. Steam the broccoli until tender, 8 to 10 minutes. Once tender, remove from the heat but keep warm until ready to serve.

3. Drain the potatoes and carrots and transfer them to the blender. Add the cashews, reserved soaking water, nutritional yeast, lemon juice, olive oil, onion powder, garlic powder, and salt. Blend until completely smooth.

4. Serve the broccoli with a pinch of salt and pepper and a few dollops of cheese sauce. Store any leftover cheese sauce in an airtight container in the fridge for 3 to 4 days.

VARIATION

If your kids don't like broccoli, try using cauliflower or another vegetable they like instead.

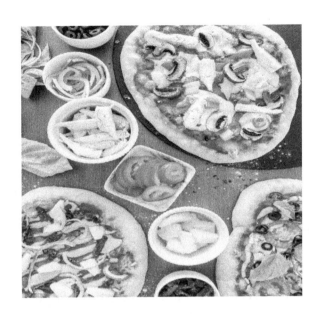

Make-Your-Own Cheese Pizza

MAKES 1 LARGE PIZZA, WITH EXTRA SAUCE

PREP TIME: **20 minutes** (not including time to make Basic Cashew Cheese Sauce or your own pizza dough)
ACTIVE TIME: **25 minutes**

pizza sauce

One 15-ounce can no-salt-added tomato sauce
One 6-ounce can no-salt-added tomato paste
1 tablespoon extra virgin olive oil
1 teaspoon dried basil
1 teaspoon dried oregano
2 pinches of garlic powder
½ cup water
Salt and black pepper to taste

pizzas
1 or more individual store-bought pizza crusts (or you can use
your favorite pizza dough recipe—most are vegan; use gluten-
free if necessary)
Basic Cashew Cheese Sauce

Assorted pizza toppings, such as sliced mushrooms, bell
peppers, red onion, artichoke hearts, chopped fresh tomatoes,
sundried tomatoes, olives, pineapple, chopped fresh basil
Sliced vegan sausage, chopped chickenless strips, or beefless
crumbles, optional

1. **To make the pizza sauce:** Combine the tomato sauce, tomato
paste, olive oil, basil, oregano, garlic powder, and water in a
medium pot and bring to a boil. Reduce to a simmer and cook,
stirring occasionally, for 15 to 20 minutes, until thickened.

2. While the sauce is simmering, follow the instructions for
your pizza crust(s) or pizza dough recipe for preheating the oven
and preparation. Prepare your toppings and place them on a tray
or set them out on the counter, getting them ready for the teens
to invade.

3. Once the oven is hot, spread sauce on top of the crust(s), leaving 1 inch around the perimeter. Drizzle or spoon the cheese sauce over the top, using as much or as little as you like. If the crusts are small enough, everyone can add make their own individual pizza. If the crusts are large, you can let each person add toppings of their choice to half of a pizza.

4. Bake the pizza(s) according to the recipe instructions. Once done, remove the pizza(s) from the oven, slice, and serve.

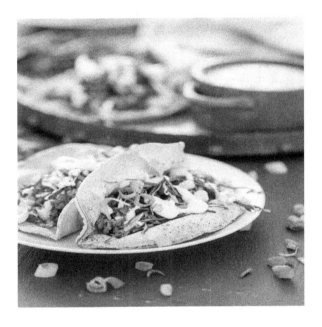

Smashed Lentil Tacos

MAKES 12 TACOS

1 quart low-sodium vegetable broth
2 cups brown lentils, rinsed and picked through
2 teaspoons ancho chile powder
2 teaspoons ground cumin
1½ teaspoons ground coriander
1 teaspoon garlic powder
1 teaspoon onion powder
½ teaspoon smoked paprika
3 tablespoons liquid aminos (or gluten-free tamari; use coconut aminos to be soy-free)
2 tablespoons lime juice
Salt and black pepper to taste
12 corn tortillas
Shredded cabbage
Guacamole or sliced avocado, optional
Salsa, optional
 Pepperjack Cheese Sauce, optional

1. In a medium pot, combine the broth, lentils, ancho chile powder, cumin, coriander, garlic powder, onion powder, and paprika. Cover the pot and bring to a boil. Once boiling, crack the lid and reduce the heat to a simmer. Let simmer until the liquid has cooked away, 15 to 20 minutes. Remove from the heat.

2. Add the liquid aminos, lime juice, salt, and pepper. Use a potato masher to smash the lentils until they slightly resemble taco meat.

3. While the lentils are cooking, you can prepare the tortillas. Heat a large frying pan, preferably cast iron, over medium heat. Place a tortilla in the pan and once the edges begin to curl up (after about 30 seconds), flip and cook for another 30 seconds. Place the heated tortilla on a plate and cover with aluminum foil. Repeat with the remaining tortillas.

4. To serve, scoop a bit of the smashed lentils onto a tortilla. Top with cabbage, and add guacamole, salsa, and/or cheese sauce (if using).

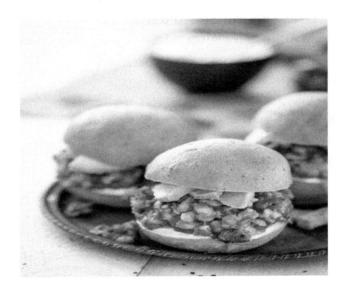

Tempeh Sloppy Joe Sliders

SERVES 8

1 teaspoon olive oil
1 medium red onion, diced
1 red bell pepper, diced
2 garlic cloves, minced
Two 8-ounce packages tempeh (soy-free if necessary), crumbled
½ cup low-sodium vegetable broth (or water)
One 15-ounce can no-salt-added crushed tomatoes
One 6-ounce can no-salt-added tomato paste
¼ cup liquid aminos (or gluten-free tamari; use coconut aminos to be soy-free)
2 tablespoons maple syrup
1½ teaspoons ground cumin
1 teaspoon dried parsley
1 teaspoon dried thyme
1 teaspoon smoked paprika
Salt and black pepper to taste
16 slider or 8 full-size vegan burger buns (gluten-free if necessary)
Vegan mayonnaise (soy-free if necessary), optional
Sliced avocado, optional

1. Heat the olive oil in a large, shallow saucepan over medium heat. Add the onion and cook until slightly translucent. Add the bell pepper and garlic and cook for a couple of minutes more, until the garlic is fragrant. Add the tempeh, broth, crushed tomatoes, tomato paste, liquid aminos, maple syrup, cumin, parsley, thyme, and paprika. Cook, stirring occasionally, until the tempeh is tender and the sauce is thick, 10 to 12 minutes. Add the salt and pepper, then remove from the heat.

2. Serve on the burger buns, slathered with mayonnaise and topped with avocado (if using).

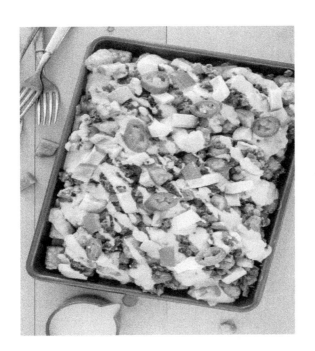

Tater Totchos

SERVES 6 TO 8

PREP TIME: **10 minutes**
ACTIVE TIME: **30 minutes**

One 32-ounce bag frozen potato tots (most are vegan, but be sure to double-check before buying)

nacho cheese sauce
1 cup chopped Yukon gold potatoes

½ cup peeled, chopped carrot
¾ cup water
¼ cup nutritional yeast
2 tablespoons tahini (gluten-free if necessary)
1½ tablespoons pickled jalapeño juice
1 tablespoon canned diced green chiles
1 tablespoon lime juice
2 teaspoons sunflower oil (or grapeseed oil), optional
1 scant tablespoon minced pickled jalapeño, optional
1 teaspoon ground cumin
½ teaspoon onion powder

beans

1 teaspoon olive oil
1 medium red onion, diced
2 garlic cloves, minced
1 red bell pepper, diced
3 cups cooked black beans (or two 15-ounce cans, rinsed and drained)
¼ cup liquid aminos (or gluten-free tamari; use coconut aminos to be soy-free)
2 teaspoons ground cumin
2 teaspoons ancho chile powder
1 teaspoon ground coriander
½ teaspoon paprika
3 tablespoons canned diced green chiles
Juice of 1 lime
Salt and black pepper to taste
Optional toppings: chopped green onions, chopped fresh tomato, pickled jalapeños, guacamole or chunks of avocado, vegan sour cream

1. Preheat the oven and bake the tots according to the package instructions.

2. While the tots are baking, **make the nacho cheese sauce:** Place the potatoes and carrots in a medium pot and cover with water. Bring to a boil and cook until the vegetables are easily pierced with a fork, 8 to 10 minutes.

3. Drain the vegetables and transfer them to your food processor. Add the water, nutritional yeast, tahini, pickled jalapeño juice, green chiles, lime juice, sunflower oil (if using), pickled jalapeño (if using), cumin, and onion powder. Process until completely smooth. Set aside.

4. **To make the beans:** Heat the olive oil in a large frying pan over medium heat. Add the onions, garlic, and red bell pepper. Sauté until the onions are slightly translucent. Add the beans, liquid aminos, cumin, ancho chile powder, coriander, and paprika. Cook until the liquid has been absorbed and the beans are heated through. Add the green chiles and lime juice and cook until the liquid has been absorbed, about 1 minute. Remove from the heat and add salt and pepper.

5. Spread out the tots on a large platter or small baking sheet. Top with the beans, then drizzle the sauce over the beans. If desired, top with green onions, tomato, jalapeños, guacamole, and/or sour cream. Serve immediately.

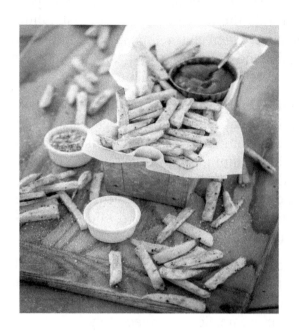

Just Fries

MAKES AS MUCH AS YOU WANT

PREP TIME: **10 minutes**
ACTIVE TIME: **10 minutes**
INACTIVE TIME: **25 minutes**

Olive oil spray
1 russet potato per person (or ½ potato per person if using as a side dish), peeled (see Tip)
Salt and black pepper to taste
Garlic powder, optional

Vegan sauces (such as ketchup, barbecue sauce, mustard, or ranch dressing; gluten-free, nut-free, and/or soy-free if necessary), for dipping

1. Preheat the oven to 450°F . Line baking sheets with aluminum foil—you can fit about 2 potatoes per baking sheet, so do the math. Lightly spray the foil with olive oil.

2. Slice each potato into similarly sized strips or wedges. It's important that they're equal size so that they cook evenly.

3. Spread out the fries on the prepared baking sheets. Spray a light coating of olive oil over the fries. Sprinkle them with salt, pepper, and garlic powder (if using). Toss to coat and rearrange the slices on the sheet so they're not touching (as much as possible). This will help them get more crispy.

4. Bake for 25 to 30 minutes, flipping them once halfway through to ensure even cooking. Once they're crispy and lightly browned on the outside but easily pierced with a fork, they're ready. Remove from the oven and serve immediately with the preferred dipping sauce(s).

TIP

You don't need to peel the potatoes if you're in a hurry, but I recommend it—it really makes a difference in flavor and texture.

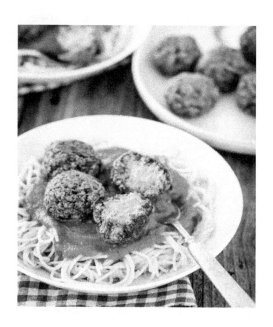

Cheese-Stuffed Meatballs

SERVES 4

PREP TIME: **15 minutes** (not including time to make Smoked Gouda Cheese Sauce and Sun-Dried Tomato Marinara Sauce)
ACTIVE TIME: **55 minutes**

1 teaspoon olive oil
½ cup chopped yellow onion
2 garlic cloves, minced
8 ounces cremini mushrooms (or button mushrooms), diced
One 15-ounce can red beans, rinsed and drained
¼ cup chopped fresh parsley
¾ cup vegan panko bread crumbs (gluten-free if necessary), plus more if needed
2 tablespoons nutritional yeast (or use more bread crumbs)

2 tablespoons liquid aminos (use coconut aminos to be soy-free)

1½ teaspoons dried basil

1½ teaspoons dried oregano

Salt and black pepper to taste

Smoked Gouda Cheese Sauce, Melty Variation (see Tip)

12 ounces spaghetti or other pasta (gluten-free if necessary), optional

4 cups Sun-Dried Tomato Marinara Sauce (or store-bought vegan marinara sauce)

1. Heat the olive oil in a large shallow saucepan over medium heat. Add the onion, garlic, and mushrooms and sauté until the mushrooms are browned and tender and the onions are translucent. Remove from the heat. Transfer to a food processor along with the beans and parsley and pulse until combined and the mixture is mostly uniform, but still a bit chunky.

2. Transfer to a large bowl along with the bread crumbs, nutritional yeast, liquid aminos, basil, oregano, salt, and pepper. Stir with a spoon or use your hands to make sure the mixture is thoroughly combined. It should stick together when squeezed. If it's still too wet, add more bread crumbs.

3. Preheat the oven to 375°F. Line a baking sheet with parchment paper or a silicone baking mat.

4. Scoop up 1 tablespoon of the mixture and roll it into a ball. Use your finger to press a little hole in the middle and shape the mixture into a tiny "bowl." Scoop ½ to ¾ teaspoon of the cheese sauce into the "bowl." Take another tablespoon of the meatball mixture, shape it into a ball, then slightly flatten it into a "dome." Place the dome on top of the meatball bowl, then use your fingers to seal the edges and shape it again into a ball. Place on the baking sheet and repeat with the remaining mixture.

5. Bake for 30 to 35 minutes, flipping once halfway through.

6. While the meatballs are in the oven, cook the pasta (if using): Bring a large pot of water to a boil and add the pasta. Cook according to the package instructions until al dente. Drain and set aside.

7. Heat the marinara sauce while the meatballs are baking.

8. Serve the meatballs on their own, covered in sauce, or on top of the pasta. Leftover meatballs and sauce will keep in an airtight container in the fridge for 3 to 4 days.

TIP

It's best to use the cheese after it's been cooked and allowed to rest for a while (or even chilled). If you have some leftover cheese from the Avocado Melt or French Onion Soup, it would be perfect for this dish since it's already thickened and firmed up a bit. If you don't have any leftover cheese, make it while you're cooking the vegetables (step 1) and let it rest or chill until ready to use.

VARIATION

You can also try using the melty variation of any of the other Basic Cashew Cheese Sauce flavors. They'll each add their own flair to the dish.

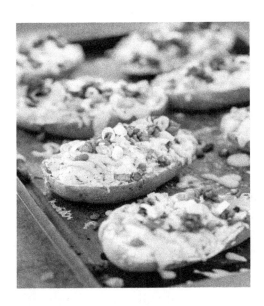

Ultimate Twice-Baked Potatoes

SERVES 4

PREP TIME: **10 minutes** (not including time to make Smoked Gouda Cheese Sauce and Quick Bacon Crumbles)
ACTIVE TIME: **20 minutes**
INACTIVE TIME: **70 minutes**

4 large russet potatoes, scrubbed and dried
Olive oil spray
8 ounces cremini mushrooms (or button mushrooms), sliced
2 tablespoons vegan butter (soy-free if necessary)
½ cup unsweetened nondairy milk (soy-free if necessary)
1 teaspoon dried thyme
1 teaspoon dried parsley
1 teaspoon onion powder
1 teaspoon garlic powder
Salt and black pepper to taste

¾ cup chopped green onions (green and white parts)

Smoked Gouda Cheese Sauce (see page

Quick Bacon Crumbles

1. Preheat the oven to 400°F. Line a baking sheet with parchment paper or a silicone baking mat. Place the potatoes on the baking sheet and stab a fork into them about four times each to create holes for steam to escape. Spray them with olive oil. Bake for 1 hour, then remove from the oven and let cool. Reduce the heat to 350°F.

2. While the potatoes are baking, heat a large frying pan over medium heat. Brown the mushroom slices, stirring occasionally, for 10 to 12 minutes. When they're done, they should be tender and golden brown. Remove from the heat and set aside.

3. When they're cool enough to handle, slice the potatoes in half lengthwise. Use a spoon to scoop out the insides of each half into a large bowl, leaving a very thin layer close to the skin to help the skin hold its shape. Mash the potatoes until mostly smooth with small chunks. Add the butter, milk, thyme, parsley, onion powder, garlic powder, salt, and pepper and stir until combined. Fold the mushrooms and ½ cup of the green onions into the mixture.

4. Scoop the mixture back into the hollowed-out skins. Return them to the oven and bake for another 20 minutes. Remove from the oven. Drizzle cashew cheese over each potato, then sprinkle the bacon crumbles and the remaining green onions on top. Serve immediately. Keep any leftovers in an airtight container in the fridge for 1 to 2 days.

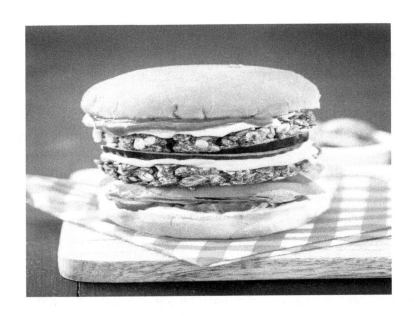

Double-Double Cheeseburgers

SERVES 4

PREP TIME: **25 minutes** (not including time to make Basic Cashew Cheese Sauce)
ACTIVE TIME: **30 minutes**   INACTIVE TIME: **20 minutes**

1 teaspoon olive oil
½ medium yellow onion, chopped
2 garlic cloves, minced
8 ounces cremini mushrooms (or button mushrooms), sliced
2 cups cooked lentils
2 tablespoons liquid aminos (or gluten-free tamari; use coconut aminos to be soy-free)
2 tablespoons nutritional yeast
1 tablespoon vegan Worcestershire sauce (gluten-free and/or soy-free if necessary), optional

1 teaspoon ground cumin
1 teaspoon dried parsley
½ teaspoon smoked paprika
½ teaspoon salt
Black pepper to taste
1 cup rolled oats (certified gluten-free if necessary), plus more if needed
½ cup quinoa flour
3 tablespoons almond flour
2 tablespoons flax meal
4 vegan burger buns (gluten-free if necessary)
Basic Cashew Cheese Sauce

Optional burger fixings: ketchup, mustard (gluten-free if necessary), vegan mayonnaise (soy-free if necessary), relish, lettuce, sliced tomatoes, sliced red onion, pickles

1. Preheat the oven to 375°F . Line a baking sheet with parchment paper or a silicone baking mat.

2. Heat the oil in a large frying pan over medium heat. Add the onion, garlic, and mushrooms and sauté until the mushrooms are tender and the onions are translucent, 4 to 5 minutes. Remove from the heat and transfer to a food processor. Add 1 cup of the lentils, the liquid aminos, nutritional yeast, Worcestershire sauce (if using), cumin, parsley, paprika, salt, and pepper. Pulse until fully combined and all pieces are similar in size.

3. Transfer to a large bowl. Add the remaining lentils, the oats, quinoa flour, almond flour, and flax meal and mix until a thick dough forms. If it's too liquidy, add more oats. If it's too dry, add water by the tablespoon until it's no longer crumbly. It should hold together without crumbling when squeezed.

4. Use your hands to form the mixture into 8 patties and place them on the baking sheet. Bake for 20 minutes, flipping once halfway through to ensure even cooking. Drizzle cheese sauce over the tops and bake for another 5 minutes.

5. To assemble, spread ketchup, mustard, mayonnaise, and/or relish on the top and bottom halves of the buns. Place some lettuce on the bottom bun and stack two patties on top. Top the patties with tomato, red onion, and/or pickles, as desired. Serve immediately. Leftover burgers will keep in an airtight container in the fridge for 4 to 5 days.

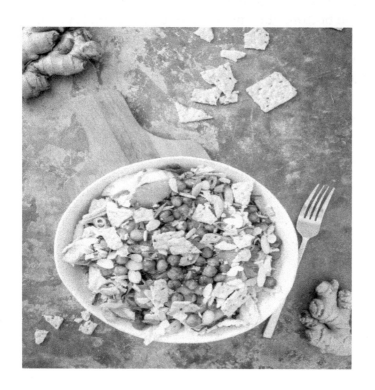

Chinese Chickpea Salad

SERVES 4 TO 6

PREP TIME: **20 minutes**
ACTIVE TIME: **15 minutes**

1 tablespoon sesame oil
3 cups cooked chickpeas (or two 15-ounce cans, rinsed and drained)
3 tablespoons gluten-free tamari (use coconut aminos to be soy-free)
4 cups shredded napa cabbage (about 1 small head)

1 cup shredded red cabbage

1 cup grated carrots (3 or 4 large carrots)

1 cup toasted sliced almonds

½ cup sliced green onions (green and white parts)

One 10-ounce can mandarin oranges (preferably packed in juice, not syrup), rinsed and drained

One 8-ounce can sliced water chestnuts, rinsed, drained, and cut in half

Crispy rice crackers, crumbled

miso ginger dressing

½ cup rice vinegar

2 tablespoons sesame oil

2 tablespoons maple syrup

1 tablespoon white soy miso (or chickpea miso)

2 teaspoons freshly grated ginger

1. Heat the sesame oil in a large shallow saucepan over medium heat. Add the chickpeas and cook for a couple of minutes. Add the tamari and cook, stirring occasionally, until the liquid has been absorbed. Set aside to cool for about 5 minutes.

2. **To make the dressing** : Stir together all the ingredients in a cup or small bowl.

3. Combine the napa cabbage, red cabbage, carrots, almonds, green onions, mandarin oranges, and water chestnuts in a large bowl. Add the chickpeas and dressing and toss until fully combined. Serve immediately, topped with crumbled rice crackers.

TIP

You can prep this ahead of time by preparing the chickpeas, the salad (without the almonds), and the dressing and storing them separately. Combine the three elements, plus the almonds, just before serving.

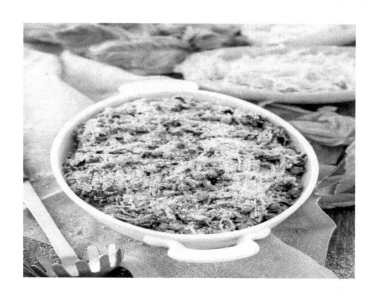

Pecan Pesto Spaghetti Squash with Peas & Kale

SERVES 4 TO 6

PREP TIME: **15 minutes** (not including time to make Pepita Parmesan)
ACTIVE TIME: **20 minutes**
INACTIVE TIME: **35 minutes**

1 medium (2-pound) spaghetti squash, halved lengthwise, seeds removed
Olive oil spray
Salt and black pepper to taste
1 teaspoon olive oil
1 shallot, chopped

1 bunch (12 to 16 ounces) kale, stems removed, chopped
1½ cups green peas (fresh or thawed frozen)
 Pepita Parmesan, optional

pecan pesto
½ cup pecan pieces
2 garlic cloves
2 cups loosely packed chopped greens of your choice (spinach, kale, or chard)
1 cup loosely packed chopped fresh basil
3 tablespoons low-sodium vegetable broth (or water)
3 tablespoons olive oil
2 tablespoons lemon juice
Salt and black pepper to taste

1. Preheat the oven to 400°F. Line a baking sheet with parchment paper or a silicone baking mat. Place the two halves of the squash on the baking sheet, cut side up. Lightly spray the top with olive oil and sprinkle with salt and pepper. Bake for 35 to 45 minutes, until the flesh is easily pulled apart with a fork. Remove from the oven and set aside to cool.

2. While the squash is roasting, **make the pesto**: Combine all the ingredients in a food processor and process until mostly smooth (teeny chunks or pieces are okay), pausing to scrape the sides as needed. Set aside until ready to use.

3. Once the squash is cool enough to touch, use a fork to tear the flesh into spaghetti-like strands.

4. Heat the olive oil in a large shallow saucepan over medium heat. Add the shallot and cook until just translucent. Add the kale, peas, and squash strands and cook, stirring occasionally, until the kale begins to wilt. Stir in the pesto sauce. Taste and add salt and pepper if necessary. Serve immediately, topped with Pepita Parmesan, if desired. Keep leftovers in an airtight container in the fridge for up to 2 days.

VARIATIONS

In the mood for pasta? Replace the spaghetti squash with cooked pasta of your choice. Rice would be another good option. In either case, pick up the recipe at step 2, making the pesto.

To make this oil-free, you can replace all the olive oil with low-sodium vegetable broth or water.

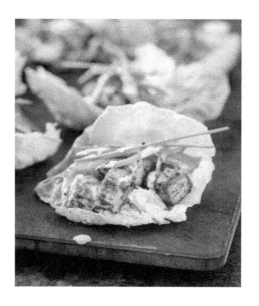

Chile-Roasted Tofu Lettuce Cups

SERVES 4

PREP TIME: **15 minutes** (not including time to make Lemon Tahini Sauce)
ACTIVE TIME: **20 minutes**
INACTIVE TIME: **45 minutes**

chile-roasted tofu

One 14-ounce block extra firm tofu, pressed for at least 1 hour (see How to Press Tofu)
¼ cup orange juice
1 tablespoon coconut oil, melted
1 tablespoon ancho chile powder
2 teaspoons maple syrup
½ teaspoon garlic powder
2 pinches of cayenne pepper
½ teaspoon salt

lettuce cups

1 large or 2 small heads butter lettuce, separated into individual leaves (see Tip)
Lemon Tahini Sauce
1 large carrot, peeled and grated
½ red bell pepper, sliced into long, thin slivers
15 to 20 chives, trimmed
White or black sesame seeds

1. **To make the tofu** : Slice the tofu horizontally so that you have two flat sheets. Dice both sheets into ½-inch cubes.

2. In a shallow baking dish, combine the orange juice, coconut oil, ancho chile powder, maple syrup, garlic powder, cayenne pepper, and salt. Add the tofu cubes and toss to coat. Marinate for about 20 minutes, tossing to recoat every 5 minutes.

3. Preheat the oven to 400°F . Line a baking sheet with parchment paper or a silicone baking mat. Spread out the tofu on the baking sheet. Bake for 25 minutes, or until the edges are crispy and browned, flipping once halfway through to ensure even cooking. Remove from the oven.

4. To serve, fill a lettuce leaf with a large spoonful of the tofu. Drizzle with tahini sauce. Top with a pinch of carrot, a couple of slivers of red bell pepper, and 1 to 2 chives. Sprinkle with sesame seeds. Leftover tofu will keep in an airtight container in the fridge for 3 to 4 days.

TIP

To prevent the lettuce leaves from tearing or falling apart when you're removing them from the head, slice the base off the head first.

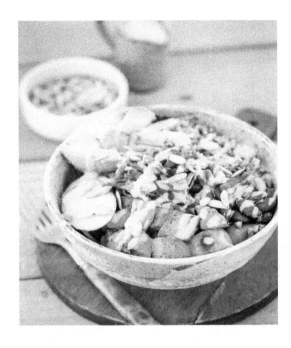

Buddha Bowl

SERVES 4

PREP TIME: **10 minutes** (not including time to make Pickled Red Cabbage & Onion Relish and Lemon Tahini Sauce or Avocado Ranch Dressing)
ACTIVE TIME: **40 minutes**

2 medium sweet potatoes or yams, peeled and chopped into 1-inch cubes
Olive oil spray
2 pinches of smoked paprika
Salt and black pepper to taste
3 cups water
1½ cups roasted buckwheat groats (kasha)
2 to 3 cups chopped spinach
1½ cups cooked, warm kidney beans (or one 15-ounce) can, rinsed and drained; or use another bean of your choice)

1 cucumber, sliced

1 avocado, pitted, peeled, and sliced

Pickled Red Cabbage & Onion Relish

Lemon Tahini Sauce or Avocado Ranch Dressing

⅓ cup toasted pepitas (pumpkin seeds)

1. Preheat the oven to 425°F. Line a baking sheet with parchment paper or a silicone baking mat. Spread out the sweet potato cubes on the pan and spray with olive oil. Add the paprika, salt, and pepper and toss to coat. Bake for 30 minutes, or until tender and browned, tossing once halfway through to ensure even cooking. Set aside to cool.

2. While the sweet potatoes are cooking, cook the buckwheat groats: Bring the water to a boil in a medium pot. Add the buckwheat groats and return to a boil. Reduce the heat, cover, and simmer until most of the water has been absorbed, 11 to 12 minutes. Remove from the heat and add salt.

3. To serve, fill each bowl with spinach, buckwheat groats, beans, sweet potato, cucumber, avocado, and cabbage relish. Drizzle with dressing and top with toasted pepitas.

VARIATION

▶ You can switch out the buckwheat groats with 3 cups cooked grain of your choice, such as rice, quinoa, millet, amaranth, or even farro (though that won't be gluten-free).

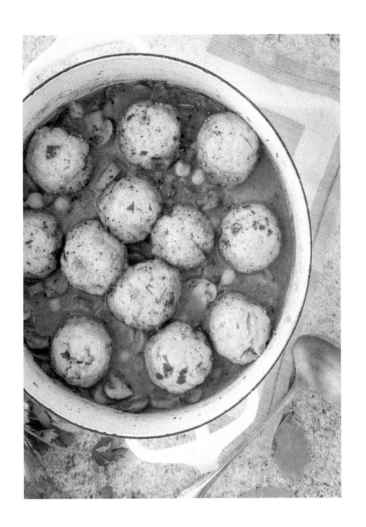

Chickpea & Dumplin' Soup

SERVES 6 TO 8

PREP TIME: **15 minutes**
ACTIVE TIME: **40 minutes** INACTIVE TIME: **15 minutes**

5 tablespoons cold vegan butter (soy-free if necessary)
1 small yellow onion, diced
4 celery stalks, sliced
3 large carrots, peeled and sliced
2 garlic cloves, minced
8 ounces cremini mushrooms (or button mushrooms), sliced
3 bay leaves
2½ teaspoons dried thyme
2 teaspoons dried rosemary
1 teaspoon dried parsley
½ teaspoon ground cumin
¼ cup oat flour (or other flour; certified gluten-free if necessary)
3 cups cooked chickpeas or two 15-ounce cans, rinsed and drained
1 quart vegetable broth
1¼ cups unbleached all-purpose flour (or gluten-free flour blend, soy-free if necessary)
½ cup fine cornmeal (certified gluten-free if necessary)
2 teaspoons baking powder

1 teaspoon baking soda

Salt and black pepper to taste

¼ teaspoon garlic powder

¼ teaspoon xanthan gum (exclude if using all-purpose flour or if your gluten-free blend includes it)

¾ cup unsweetened nondairy milk (nut-free and/or soy-free if necessary)

2 tablespoons chopped fresh parsley

1. Melt 1 tablespoon of the butter over medium heat in a large Dutch oven or pot (choose a wide one to give you more dumpling surface area). Add the onion, celery, carrot, and garlic and cook for about 3 minutes. Add the mushrooms and cook for 3 minutes more, stirring occasionally. Stir in the bay leaves, 2 teaspoons of the thyme, the rosemary, dried parsley, and cumin and cook for 1 minute. Add the oat flour and stir until the flour is no longer visible. Add the chickpeas and broth, bring to a boil, then reduce to a simmer. Cover and cook for about 10 minutes, stirring every few minutes to prevent sticking.

2. In a large bowl, combine the all-purpose flour, cornmeal, baking powder, baking soda, ½ teaspoon salt, the garlic powder, and xanthan gum (if using). Add the remaining butter and use a pastry cutter or a fork to cut the butter into the flour mixture until you have a coarse meal, similar to the texture of wet sand. In a cup or small bowl, combine the milk and fresh parsley. Pour over the flour mixture. Stir until you have a thick dough.

3. Uncover the pot and remove the bay leaves. Add salt and pepper. Drop the dough into the soup in 8 to 10 large spoonfuls. Space the dumplings evenly, keeping in mind that they'll expand. Cover and cook for 15 minutes more, or until the dumplings are solid. Sprinkle with more pepper. Serve immediately. Leftovers will keep in an airtight container in the fridge for 2 to 3 days.

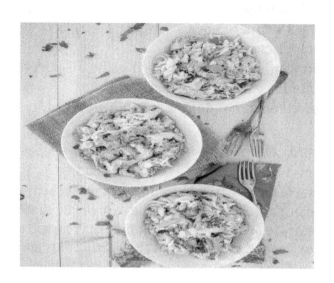

Shiitake Stroganoff

SERVES 4

PREP TIME: **30 minutes**
ACTIVE TIME: **25 minutes**

12 ounces spiral pasta (gluten-free if necessary)
One 12-ounce vacuum-packed block extra firm silken tofu
3 tablespoons lemon juice
1 tablespoon unsweetened nondairy milk (nut-free if necessary)
2 teaspoons white wine vinegar
1 teaspoon olive oil
4 shallots, chopped

1 garlic clove, minced
1 pound shiitake mushrooms, stemmed and sliced (see Variation)
½ cup vegan white wine (or low-sodium vegetable broth)
2 teaspoons nutritional yeast, optional
1 teaspoon paprika
1 cup chopped fresh parsley
Salt and black pepper to taste

1. Bring a large pot of water to a boil and add the pasta. Cook according to the package instructions until al dente. Drain and set aside.

2. Combine the tofu, lemon juice, milk, and vinegar in a food processor and process until smooth. Set aside.

3. Heat the olive oil in a large shallow saucepan over medium heat. Add the shallots and garlic and sauté until the shallots are almost translucent.

4. Add the mushrooms and cook, stirring occasionally, until the mushrooms are tender, 10 to 12 minutes. Add the wine and cook until the liquid has been absorbed. Stir in the nutritional yeast and paprika.

5. Add the reserved tofu mixture and cook until heated through. Add the parsley, salt, and pepper. Fold in the pasta and serve immediately. Refrigerate any leftovers in an airtight container for up to 3 days.

VARIATION

➤ You can use other types of mushrooms, or even a mixture of mushrooms, to replace the shiitakes.

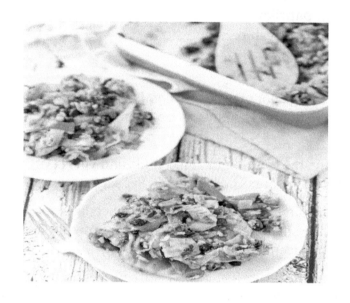

Unstuffed Cabbage Rolls

SERVES 8

PREP TIME: **30 minutes** (not including time to cook brown rice)
ACTIVE TIME: **20 minutes**
INACTIVE TIME: **30 minutes**

Olive oil spray
1 large (2- to 3-pound) head cabbage, quartered and cored
1 teaspoon olive oil
1 medium sweet onion, diced

2 garlic cloves, minced
1 red bell pepper, diced
3 cups cooked black beans or two 15-ounce cans, rinsed and
drained
One 15-ounce can no-salt-added fire-roasted diced tomatoes
2 tablespoons no-salt-added tomato paste
2 tablespoons liquid aminos (or gluten-free tamari; use
coconut aminos to be soy-free)
1 teaspoon dried parsley
1 teaspoon dried oregano
½ teaspoon ground cumin
½ teaspoon paprika
1½ cups cooked brown rice (or other grain)
2 tablespoons nutritional yeast
2 tablespoons lemon juice
Salt and black pepper to taste

1. Preheat the oven to 375°F. Lightly spray a 9 × 13-inch baking
dish with olive oil.

2. Chop each cabbage quarter into 1-inch strips. Set aside.

3. Heat the olive oil in a large shallow saucepan over medium
heat. Add the onion and garlic and sauté until the onion is just
becoming translucent.

4. Add the bell pepper, black beans, tomatoes with their juice,
tomato paste, liquid aminos, parsley, oregano, cumin, and
paprika. Cover and cook, stirring occasionally, until the bell
pepper is tender.

5. Add the cabbage, cover again, and cook until the cabbage is soft. Stir in the rice and cook until heated through. Add the nutritional yeast, lemon juice, salt, and pepper. Remove from the heat.

6. Transfer to the baking dish and bake, uncovered, for 25 minutes. Let cool for a few minutes before serving. Leftovers will keep in an airtight container in the fridge for 4 to 5 days.

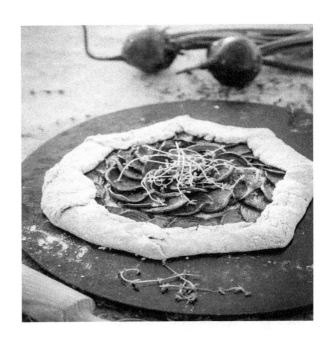

Balsamic-Roasted Beet & Cheese Galette

SERVES 4

PREP TIME: **20 minutes** (not including time to make Mixed
Herb Cheese Sauce)
ACTIVE TIME: **70 minutes**
INACTIVE TIME: **40 minutes**

crust

¼ cup unsweetened nondairy milk (soy-free if necessary)
3 tablespoons aquafaba

71

1½ cups unbleached all-purpose flour (or gluten-free flour blend, soy-free if necessary), plus more for the work surface
1 tablespoon coconut sugar
½ teaspoon salt
½ teaspoon baking soda
½ teaspoon xanthan gum (exclude if using all-purpose flour or if your gluten-free blend includes it)
8 tablespoons very cold vegan butter (soy-free if necessary; see Tip)

filling

Olive oil spray
2 medium red beets, peeled and very thinly sliced (see Tip)
2 medium golden beets, peeled and very thinly sliced (see Tip)
6 tablespoons balsamic vinegar
2 tablespoons coconut sugar
Salt and black pepper to taste
Mixed Herb Cheese Sauce, Spread Variation
Fresh thyme leaves

1. **To make the crust** : In a small cup or bowl, combine the milk and aquafaba. Set aside.

2. In a large bowl, whisk together the flour, coconut sugar, salt, baking soda, and xanthan gum (if using). Using a pastry cutter or fork, cut the butter into the flour until it's evenly incorporated and the mixture resembles small peas. Slowly pour in the milk mixture until the dough just comes together. Turn the dough out onto a floured surface and work it into a roughly 2-inch-thick disk. Wrap the dough in plastic wrap and refrigerate for at least 30 minutes. (This can be done 1 to 3 days in advance.)

3. While the dough is chilling, **make the filling** : Preheat the oven to 400°F . Lightly spray two 9 × 13-inch (23 × 33-cm) baking dishes with olive oil. Spread out the red beet slices in one dish and the golden beets in the other (you can do them all in one, but the red beets will stain the golden beets). Drizzle 3 tablespoons of the vinegar over each set of beets, then add 1 tablespoon coconut sugar per dish and top with salt and pepper. Toss to coat, then spread out the slices again (it's okay if they overlap). Bake for about 15 minutes, flipping once halfway through. The beets will be undercooked, which is okay. Remove them from the oven and set aside.

4. Reduce the temperature to 350°F. Line a baking sheet, pizza pan, or pizza stone with parchment paper or a silicone baking mat.

5. Once the dough has chilled for at least 30 minutes, remove it from the refrigerator. Remove the plastic wrap (set it aside for now) and place the dough on a floured surface. Turn it over so both sides are lightly floured. If the dough is hard, knead it lightly with your hands to make it pliable. If it's too dry and begins to crack, sprinkle with a couple of drops of water. Lay the plastic wrap on top of the dough and use a rolling pin to roll it out until it's a circle about 10 inches in diameter and ¼ inch (6 mm) thick. Gently transfer the dough to the prepared baking sheet, pan, or stone. (I do this by scooting a thin, rimless baking sheet under the dough to transport it to the other baking sheet; a pizza peel may also work.)

6. Spread the cheese on top of the dough, leaving about 1½ inches around the perimeter. Lay the beet slices on top of the cheese. You can lay them out willy-nilly or in a pretty pattern— your choice. If there is any liquid in the baking dish, pour it over the beets. Fold the edges of the dough over the beets.

7. Bake for 35 to 40 minutes, until the dough is golden brown. Remove from the oven, slice, and serve topped with fresh thyme. Leftovers will keep in an airtight container in the fridge for up to 2 days.

TIP

About 10 minutes before using vegan butter, stick it in the freezer so it gets extra cold.

When slicing your beets, it's best to use a mandoline to get superthin slices.

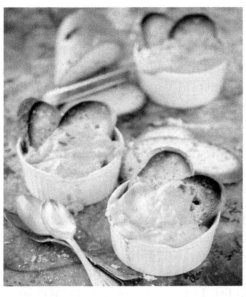

French Onion Soup

SERVES 6

PREP TIME: 30 minutes (not including time to make Smoky Gouda Cheese Sauce)

ACTIVE TIME: 60 minutes

4 tablespoons vegan butter (soy-free if necessary)
6 medium yellow onions, halved and very thinly sliced
2 garlic cloves, minced
1 tablespoon fresh thyme leaves
2 bay leaves
1 cup vegan dry white wine
2 tablespoons oat flour (certified gluten-free if necessary)
2 quarts low-sodium vegetable broth
1 tablespoon nutritional yeast, optional
Salt and black pepper to taste
1 vegan baguette, sliced (gluten-free if necessary)
Smoked Gouda Cheese Sauce, "Melty" Variation (see Tip)
Chopped fresh parsley, optional

1. Melt the butter in a large pot or Dutch oven over medium heat. Add the onions and cook for 20 to 25 minutes, stirring every so often, until browned and caramelized. Add the garlic, thyme, and bay leaves and cook for 2 to 3 minutes more, until the garlic is fragrant. Add the wine and cook, stirring occasionally, until the liquid has been absorbed. Add the oat flour and cook, stirring constantly, until the flour is no longer visible, about 2 minutes.

2. Add the broth and bring to a boil. Reduce the heat and simmer for about 15 minutes, until thickened. Add the nutritional yeast (if using), salt, and pepper. Remove from the heat and discard the bay leaves.

3. Preheat the oven broiler. Arrange six small ovenproof bowls or ramekins on a baking sheet. Pour the soup into the bowls. Place 1 or 2 baguette slices on top of the soup. Spoon the cheese sauce over the bread. Place the baking sheet with the bowls under the broiler. Broil for 3 to 4 minutes, until the cheese is browned and bubbly. Remove from the heat and sprinkle with parsley (if using). Serve immediately. Leftover soup will keep in an airtight container in the fridge for 2 to 3 days.

TIP

Heating the cheese sauce will take 5 to 7 minutes, so I suggest preparing it while the soup is simmering.

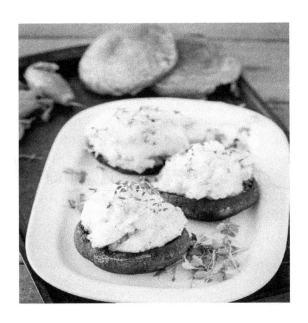

Truffled Mashed Potato–Stuffed Portobellos

SERVES 4

PREP TIME: **25 minutes** (not including time to cook mashed potatoes)
ACTIVE TIME: **30 minutes**
INACTIVE TIME: **20 minutes**

4 large portobello mushrooms
2 teaspoons vegan butter (soy-free if necessary)
2 shallots, diced
1 garlic clove, minced
2 teaspoons fresh thyme leaves, plus more for garnish
Olive oil spray
Salt and black pepper to taste

½ batch Truffled Mashed Potatoes (see Tip)

1. Preheat the oven to 375°F . Line a baking sheet with parchment paper or a silicone baking mat.

2. Remove the stems from the portobellos and set aside the caps. Dice the stems into ½-inch pieces. Melt the butter in a large frying pan, preferably cast iron, over medium heat. Add the shallots, garlic, mushroom stems, and thyme. Cook for about 5 minutes, stirring occasionally, until the mushrooms are tender. Remove from the heat.

3. Spray the tops of the portobello caps with olive oil and place gill side up on the baking sheet. Sprinkle with salt and pepper, then divide the stem mixture among them. Scoop heaping mounds of mashed potatoes on top. Bake for 20 minutes, or until the mashed potatoes are golden. Serve immediately, garnished with more thyme leaves.

VARIATION

To fancy up this dish, mash the potatoes until they're very smooth and transfer them to a pastry bag. Pipe the mashed potatoes into the mushroom caps as if you were icing a cupcake. Proceed with the instructions from there.

TIP

If you don't already have the mashed potatoes on hand, prepare them while you preheat the oven.

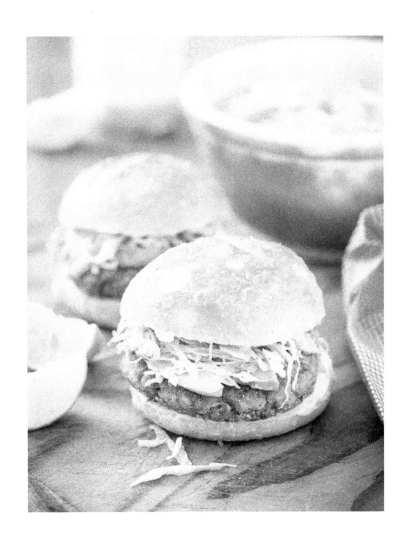

Fillet o' Chickpea Sandwich with Tartar Sauce Slaw

MAKES 6 SANDWICHES

PREP TIME: **25 minutes** (not including time to cook brown rice and make Basic Cashew Cheese Sauce)
ACTIVE TIME: **50 minutes**
INACTIVE TIME: **2 hours**

tartar sauce
½ cup raw cashews, soaked in warm water for 1 hour and drained, water reserved
¼ cup reserved soaking water
¼ cup vegan mayonnaise (soy-free if necessary)
¼ cup lemon juice
1 tablespoon caper brine
1 teaspoon dried dill

slaw
3 cups shredded cabbage
1 cup grated carrot

chickpea fillets
1½ cups cooked chickpeas (or one 15-ounce can, rinsed and drained)
1 tablespoon liquid aminos (use coconut aminos to be soy-free)
One 14- to 15-ounce can artichoke hearts, rinsed and drained

1 cup cooked brown rice

¼ cup + 1 tablespoon chickpea flour, plus more if needed

1 tablespoon Old Bay Seasoning

½ to 1 teaspoon kelp granules

½ teaspoon dried dill

Salt and black pepper to taste

1½ cups vegan bread crumbs (gluten-free if necessary)

Vegetable oil for pan-frying

sandwiches

Basic Cashew Cheese Sauce

6 vegan sandwich rolls or burger buns (gluten-free if necessary), split horizontally

Sliced avocado

1. **To make the tartar sauce** : Combine the tartar sauce ingredients in a food processor or blender and process until smooth.

2. **To make the slaw** : Combine the shredded cabbage and carrots in a large bowl and add ½ cup of the tartar sauce. Mix until fully combined and chill for at least 1 hour. Transfer the remaining tartar sauce to a small bowl and refrigerate until needed.

3. **To make the chickpea fillets** : Heat a large frying pan, preferably cast iron, over medium heat. Add the chickpeas and cook for a couple of minutes. Add the liquid aminos and cook for 5 to 7 minutes, stirring occasionally, until the liquid has been absorbed. Remove from the heat. Use a fork or pastry cutter to gently mash the chickpeas. You only have to mash them a bit; you still want them a little chunky.

4. Place the artichoke hearts in a food processor and pulse 5 to 7 times, until the artichokes are broken down into little pieces but not mushy.

5. Combine the chickpeas, artichokes, rice, and chickpea flour in a large bowl. Use your hands to mash the mixture until it's fully combined and will hold together when you squeeze it. If it doesn't hold together, add more chickpea flour by the tablespoon until it holds. Add the Old Bay, kelp granules to taste, the dill, salt, and pepper and mix until combined.

6. Line a baking sheet with parchment paper or a silicone baking mat. Line a plate with paper towels to drain the cooked fillets.

7. Pour the bread crumbs into a shallow bowl. Divide the chickpea mixture into six equal portions. One at a time, shape each into the fillet shape of your choice (round, square, rectangle), place in the bread crumbs, and gently flip until all sides are covered. Gently shake off the excess crumbs and place on the prepared baking sheet.

8. Heat a large frying pan over medium heat. Add oil until the bottom of the pan is thinly coated. Once the oil begins to shimmer, add 2 or 3 fillets. Cook for 2 to 3 minutes on each side, until both sides are golden. Transfer the fillets to the paper-towel-lined plate to drain the excess oil. Cover with a clean kitchen cloth to keep warm while you repeat with the remaining filets (adding more oil to the pan if necessary).

9. **To assemble each sandwich** : Spread cheese on the bottom half of a roll and spread tartar sauce on the top half. Place a fillet on top of the cheese sauce, then add some avocado slices, a pile of slaw, and cover with the top half of the roll. Serve immediately. If you plan to eat the sandwich later, store it in an airtight container and refrigerate for up 5 hours. Leftover fillets will keep in an airtight container in the fridge for 3 to 4 days.

The Portobello Philly Reuben

MAKES 4 SANDWICHES

PREP TIME: **15 minutes** (not including time to make Smoked Gouda Cheese Sauce)
ACTIVE TIME: **20 minutes** INACTIVE TIME: **10 minutes**

Russian dressing

⅓ cup vegan mayonnaise (soy-free if necessary)
1 tablespoon ketchup
1 tablespoon no-salt-added tomato paste
2 teaspoons red wine vinegar
1 teaspoon dried dill
½ teaspoon smoked paprika
2 to 3 tablespoons sweet pickle relish

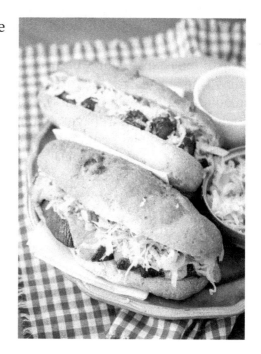

sandwiches
4 portobello mushroom caps
Olive oil spray
2 tablespoons liquid aminos (or gluten-free tamari; use coconut aminos to be soy-free)
2 tablespoons vegan Worcestershire sauce (gluten-free and/or soy-free if necessary)
Black pepper to taste
4 vegan sandwich rolls (gluten-free if necessary), split horizontally
Smoked Gouda Cheese Sauce, Melty Variation
Loads of sauerkraut

1. **To make the Russian dressing** : Stir together the mayonnaise, ketchup, tomato paste, vinegar, dill, and paprika in a small bowl. Add relish to taste. Chill until ready to use.

2. **To make the sandwiches** : Preheat the oven to 425°F. Line a baking sheet with parchment paper or a silicone baking mat. Lightly spray the top and bottom of each portobello cap with olive oil and place on the baking sheet gill side up.

3. In a small cup or bowl, mix together the liquid aminos and Worcestershire sauce. Drizzle over the mushrooms, then sprinkle with pepper. Bake for 10 minutes. Remove from the oven and let cool for a few minutes. Slice the mushrooms on a bias into ½-inch strips. Heat the cheese sauce and keep warm.

4. Preheat the broiler. Arrange the rolls on the baking sheet, cut side up. Lay portobello strips on the bottom halves. Spread or drop cheese sauce on top of the mushrooms. Place under the broiler for 1 to 2 minutes, until the cheese is golden and the bread is toasted.

5. Add a pile of sauerkraut onto the cheesy half of each sandwich, then spread Russian dressing on the top half of each roll. Place the top half on top of the sandwich and serve immediately.

BBQ Pulled Jackfruit Sandwich

MAKES 4 SANDWICHES

PREP TIME: **10 minutes** (not including time to make Creamy, Crunchy Coleslaw)
ACTIVE TIME: **20 minutes**
INACTIVE TIME: **20 minutes**

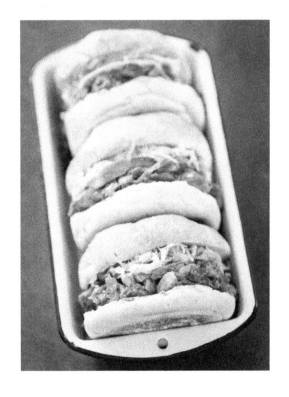

BBQ jackfruit

One 20-ounce can jackfruit (packed in brine or water, not syrup)

1 teaspoon olive oil

½ sweet onion, chopped

1 garlic clove, minced

½ teaspoon ground cumin

½ teaspoon smoked paprika

¾ cup vegan barbecue sauce (homemade or store-bought)

1 to 2 tablespoons sriracha

2 teaspoons arrowroot powder

Salt and black pepper to taste

sandwiches

4 vegan sandwich rolls or burger buns (gluten-free if necessary), split horizontally

Creamy, Crunchy Coleslaw

Sliced avocado, optional

1. Preheat the oven to 400°F. Line a baking sheet with parchment paper or a silicone baking mat.

2. Rinse and drain the jackfruit. Use two forks or your fingers to pull it apart into shreds, so that it somewhat resembles pulled meat. It will fall apart even more when you cook it.

3. Heat the oil in a large shallow saucepan over medium heat. Add the onion and garlic and sauté until the onion is translucent. Add the jackfruit, cumin, and paprika and cook, stirring occasionally, for about 5 minutes. Add salt and pepper.

4. In a cup or small bowl, stir together the barbecue sauce, sriracha, and arrowroot powder. Add to the jackfruit. Cook for 1 minute.

5. Spread out the jackfruit on the prepared baking sheet. Bake for 20 minutes, stirring once halfway through, until sauce is thick and sticky.

6. **To assemble the sandwich** : Open a roll on a plate. Place avocado slices (if using) on the bottom half. Scoop a heap of the jackfruit on top, then top the jackfruit with a pile of coleslaw. Place the other half of the roll on top and serve immediately. Leftover jackfruit will keep in an airtight container in the fridge for 3 to 4 days.

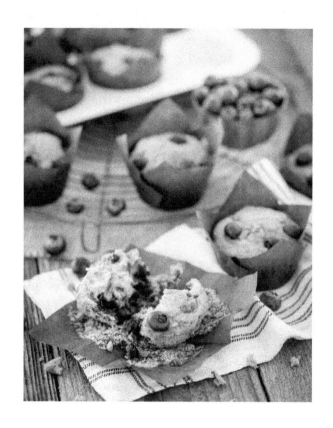

Blueberry-Banana Muffins

MAKES 12 MUFFINS

PREP TIME: **10 minutes**
ACTIVE TIME: **25 minutes**
INACTIVE TIME: **20 minutes**

¾ cup nondairy milk (nut-free and/or soy-free if necessary)
1 teaspoon apple cider vinegar
2 cups oat flour (certified gluten-free if necessary)
⅓ cup sweet white rice flour
1 tablespoon cornstarch (or arrowroot powder)
1 tablespoon baking powder
½ teaspoon ground cinnamon
½ teaspoon salt
2 ripe (very speckled) medium bananas, mashed
⅓ cup maple syrup
2 tablespoons coconut oil, melted
1 tablespoon flax meal
1 teaspoon vanilla extract
1 cup fresh blueberries (see Tip)
⅓ cup coconut sugar

1. Preheat the oven to 350°F. Line a 12-cup muffin tin with paper or silicone liners.

2. Combine the milk and vinegar in a cup or small bowl. Set aside.

3. Combine the oat flour, rice flour, cornstarch, baking powder, cinnamon, and salt in a large bowl and whisk until thoroughly combined.

4. Combine the bananas, maple syrup, coconut oil, flax meal, and vanilla in a medium bowl and add the milk mixture. Stir until combined. Add the wet ingredients to the dry ingredients and stir together until combined. Fold in the blueberries and sugar.

5. Pour the batter into the muffin tin. Bake for 23 to 25 minutes, until the tops are golden and firm. Let the muffins cool in the tin for about 5 minutes before transferring to a cooling rack. Cool completely before serving. Leftovers will keep in the fridge or at room temperature for 3 to 4 days.

TIP

You can use frozen blueberries instead of fresh, but to prevent them from bleeding, make sure to keep them in the freezer until just before you use them.

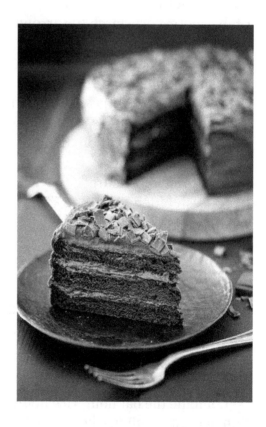

Chocolate Layer Cake

SERVES 12

PREP TIME: **15 minutes**
ACTIVE TIME: **40 minutes**
INACTIVE TIME: **60 minutes**

chocolate cake

Vegan cooking spray (or vegan butter; soy-free if necessary)
2¼ cups unsweetened vanilla nondairy milk (nut-free and/or soy-free if necessary)
3 tablespoons apple cider vinegar
3 cups white rice flour
1½ cups cocoa powder
¼ cup + 2 tablespoons oat flour (certified gluten-free if necessary)
¼ cup + 2 tablespoons coconut sugar
1 tablespoon baking powder
1 tablespoon baking soda
1½ teaspoons salt
1 cup maple syrup
12 tablespoons vegan butter (soy-free if necessary), melted
½ cup + 1 tablespoon aquafaba
1 tablespoon vanilla extract

frosting

1 cup vegan chocolate chips (or chunks)
3 cups pitted Medjool dates
1 cup unsweetened vanilla nondairy milk (nut-free and/or soy-free if necessary)
¼ cup cocoa powder
1 teaspoon vanilla extract
½ teaspoon salt
Vegan chocolate shavings, optional

1. Preheat the oven to 350°F. Lightly spray three 9-inch cake pans with cooking spray or grease them with a bit of butter.

2. **To make the cake** : Combine the milk and vinegar in a medium bowl. Set aside.

3. Whisk together the rice flour, cocoa powder, oat flour, sugar, baking powder, baking soda, and salt in a large bowl.

4. Add the maple syrup, butter, aquafaba, and vanilla to the milk mixture and whisk until combined. Add the wet ingredients to the dry ingredients and stir until thoroughly combined and smooth.

5. Distribute the batter evenly among the three pans. Bake for 35 to 40 minutes, until a toothpick inserted into the center comes out clean. Let the layers cool in the pans for about 30 minutes. Run a knife around the inside edge of the cake pans and gently transfer the layers to cooling racks to let them cool completely.

6. Once the layers come out of the oven, **make the frosting** : Melt the chocolate chips in a double boiler or a heatproof bowl on top a pot of boiling water, stirring occasionally, until smooth. Remove from the heat. Combine the dates and milk in a food processor and process until smooth. Add the melted chocolate, cocoa powder, vanilla, and salt and process until smooth. Transfer the frosting to a jar and refrigerate for at least 30 minutes, or until ready to use.

7. Once the frosting has chilled and thickened, place one of the layers on a plate or serving dish. Using a thin silicone spatula or a butter knife, evenly spread a layer of frosting on top. Place another layer on top of the frosting. Evenly spread frosting on the top of the second layer, then top with the third layer. Spread the rest of the frosting evenly over the top and around the sides until the entire cake is covered. Top with chocolate shavings, if desired. Slice and serve. The cake will keep, covered, at room temperature or in the fridge for 3 to 4 days.

▶ To make 12 cupcakes, divide the quantity of the cake ingredients by three and the frosting ingredients by two. Line the cups of a 12-cup muffin tin with paper or silicone liners and distribute the batter evenly among the cups. Bake for 18 to 20 minutes, until a toothpick inserted into the center comes out almost clean. Let the cupcakes cool in the tin for 30 minutes before transferring them to the cooling rack. Cool completely before frosting.

TIP

▶ The frosted cake will gain moisture and firmness if refrigerated in an airtight container overnight.

Peanut Butter Oatmeal Cookies

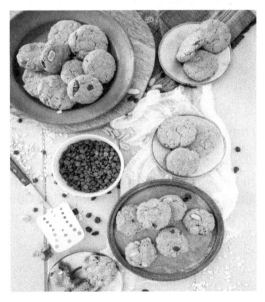

MAKES 30 COOKIES

PREP TIME: **10 minutes**
ACTIVE TIME: **20 minutes**
INACTIVE TIME: **10 minutes**

1 cup unbleached all-purpose flour (or gluten-free flour blend, soy-free if necessary)
1 cup rolled oats (certified gluten-free if necessary)

1 teaspoon baking soda
1 teaspoon ground cinnamon
½ teaspoon salt
½ teaspoon xanthan gum (exclude if using all-purpose flour or if your gluten-free blend includes it)
¼ teaspoon ground nutmeg
1 cup unsalted, unsweetened natural peanut butter
½ cup maple syrup
⅓ cup unsweetened applesauce (or mashed banana)
¼ cup coconut oil, melted
¼ cup coconut sugar, optional
1 teaspoon vanilla extract

Optional add-ins: ½ cup raisins, chopped peanuts, and/or vegan chocolate chips

1. Preheat the oven to 350°F. Line two baking sheets with parchment paper or silicone baking mats.

2. In a large bowl, whisk together the flour, oats, baking soda, cinnamon, salt, xanthan gum (if using), and nutmeg until fully incorporated.

3. In a medium bowl, combine the peanut butter, maple syrup, applesauce, coconut oil, coconut sugar (if using), and vanilla. Stir until combined.

4. Add the wet ingredients to the dry ingredients and stir until combined. If you're using add-ins, fold them in.

5. Scoop a heaping tablespoon of dough out of the bowl, roll it in your hands to make a perfect ball, and place it on the baking sheet. Repeat with the remaining dough, spacing the balls 1½ inches apart. Use your fingers to gently flatten each ball just a bit.

6. Bake for 10 to 12 minutes, until firm and slightly golden along the bottom. Let the cookies cool on the baking sheets for about 5 minutes before transferring them to a cooling rack. Cool completely before serving. The cookies will keep stored in an airtight container (in the fridge if the weather is warm) for 3 to 4 days.

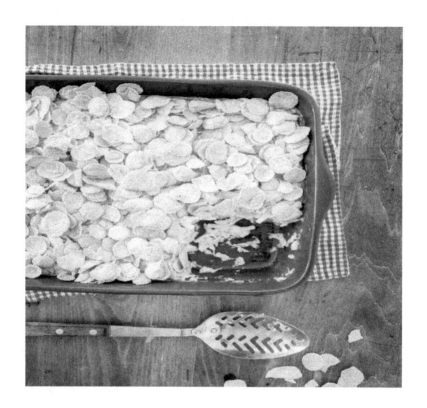

Hash Brown Casserole (aka Company Potatoes)

SERVES 6 TO 8

PREP TIME: **25 minutes** (not including time to make Cream of Mushroom Soup)
ACTIVE TIME: **5 minutes**
INACTIVE TIME: **35 minutes**

Olive oil spray
Cream of Mushroom Soup

¾ cup plain coconut yogurt (or soy yogurt; preferably unsweetened)

½ cup nutritional yeast

¾ cup sauerkraut

½ cup chopped yellow onion

One 20-ounce package frozen hash browns, thawed

3½ cups vegan cornflakes (certified gluten-free if necessary)

4 tablespoons vegan butter (soy-free if necessary), melted

1. Preheat the oven to 350°F. Lightly spray a 9 × 13-inch baking dish with olive oil.

2. In a large bowl, stir together the soup, yogurt, and nutritional yeast. Stir in the sauerkraut, onion, and hash browns. Spread out the mixture in the prepared baking dish. Bake for 15 minutes.

3. While the casserole is baking, combine the cornflakes and melted butter in a medium bowl. After the casserole has baked for 15 minutes, spread the cornflakes over the top and return to the oven. Bake for 15 minutes more, or until the casserole is bubbly and the cornflakes are crispy and golden. Remove from the oven and let rest for 5 minutes before serving. Leftovers will keep in an airtight container in the fridge for up to 4 days.

Roasted Carrot & Wild Mushroom Ragout

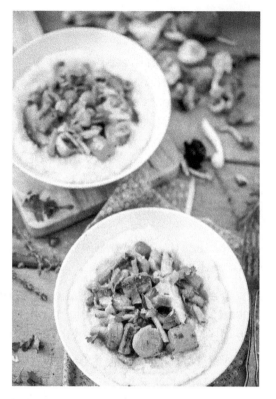

SERVES 4

PREP TIME: **30 minutes** (not including time to make polenta)
ACTIVE TIME: **40 minutes**

8 large carrots, peeled and chopped into 1-inch pieces
Olive oil spray
1 teaspoon dried thyme
1 teaspoon dried parsley
Salt and black pepper to taste
3 cups water
2 ounces dried mushrooms (porcini or a mixed variety)
2 tablespoons vegan butter (soy-free if necessary)
½ red onion, chopped
2 garlic cloves, minced
1 tablespoon chopped fresh rosemary
1 tablespoon chopped fresh thyme
8 ounces button mushrooms (or cremini mushrooms), halved
8 ounces wild mushrooms (shiitake, chanterelle, oyster, morel, lobster, etc.; see Tip), sliced
2 tablespoons oat flour (certified gluten-free if necessary)

½ cup vegan red wine
3 tablespoons lemon juice
Cooked polenta or other grain or pasta
Chopped fresh parsley, optional

1. Preheat the oven to 425°F (220°C). Line a baking sheet with parchment paper or a silicone baking mat. Spread out the carrots on the sheet and lightly spray with olive oil. Sprinkle with the dried thyme, dried parsley, and salt and pepper. Toss to coat. Roast for 25 minutes, or until caramelized and tender. Set aside until ready to use.

2. Once the carrots are in the oven, bring the water to a boil in a medium pot, then remove from the heat. Add the dried mushrooms and set aside.

3. Melt the butter in a large shallow saucepan over medium heat. Add the onion and sauté until translucent. Add the garlic, rosemary, and fresh thyme and cook until fragrant, about 2 minutes. Add the button and wild mushrooms. Use a slotted spoon to scoop the rehydrated mushrooms from the water into the pan (do not discard the water). Cook for 8 to 10 minutes, stirring occasionally, until the mushrooms are tender but still hold their shape.

4. Add the oat flour and cook, stirring constantly, until the flour is fully incorporated. Add the wine and cook, stirring frequently, until the liquid has reduced. Add ½ cup of the reserved mushroom soaking water, bring to a boil, then reduce to a simmer. Cook for about 5 minutes, until most of the liquid has been absorbed.

5. Add the carrots, lemon juice, salt, and pepper and remove from the heat. Serve over creamy polenta, garnished with fresh parsley, if desired. Leftovers will keep in an airtight container in the fridge for 2 to 3 days.

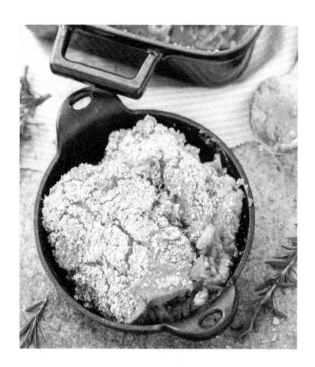

Sweet Potato Shepherd's Pie

SERVES 6

PREP TIME: **15 minutes** (not including time to make Pepita Parmesan)
ACTIVE TIME: **35 minutes**
INACTIVE TIME: **15 minutes**

Olive oil spray

topping

2 pounds sweet potatoes or yams, peeled and chopped
2 tablespoons unsweetened nondairy milk (nut-free and/or soy-free if necessary)

2 tablespoons olive oil
1 tablespoon nutritional yeast, optional
½ teaspoon garlic powder
Salt and black pepper to taste

Pepita Parmesan

Chopped fresh rosemary

filling
1 teaspoon olive oil
1 red onion, diced
2 garlic cloves, minced
2 large carrots, peeled and chopped
3 celery stalks, chopped
3 cups cooked great Northern beans (or two 15-ounce cans), rinsed and drained)
8 ounces cremini mushrooms (or button mushrooms), sliced
1 tablespoon chopped fresh rosemary
1 tablespoon chopped fresh thyme
½ cup low-sodium vegetable broth
2 tablespoons liquid aminos (or gluten-free tamari; use coconut aminos to be soy-free)
2 tablespoons no-salt-added tomato paste
¼ cup chopped sun-dried tomatoes (rehydrated in water and drained, if necessary)
¼ cup chopped pitted green olives
1 tablespoon lemon juice
Salt and black pepper to taste

1. Preheat the oven to 400°F . Lightly spray an 8-inch square or 10-inch round baking dish with olive oil. Alternatively, if you have a shallow Dutch oven or large cast-iron skillet, you can use that to cook the filling, then bake the casserole.

2. **To make the topping** : Place the sweet potatoes in a medium pot and cover with water. Bring to a boil and cook for 8 to 10 minutes, until easily pierced with a fork. Remove from the heat and drain. Add the milk, olive oil, nutritional yeast (if using), and garlic powder and mash until smooth. Alternatively, you can use a hand mixer or food processor. Once smooth, add salt and pepper.

3. While the sweet potatoes are boiling, **make the filling** : Heat the olive oil in a large, shallow saucepan that can go into the oven (or a Dutch oven or cast-iron skillet) over medium heat. Add the onion and garlic and sauté for 2 to 3 minutes, until the onion just becomes translucent. Add the carrots and celery and cook for another 3 minutes. Add the beans, mushrooms, rosemary, and thyme. Cook for about 5 minutes, stirring occasionally.

4. Combine the broth, liquid aminos, and tomato paste in a cup or small bowl and stir until combined. Add to the vegetables with the sun-dried tomatoes and olives and cook for about 5 minutes more. Remove from the heat and add the lemon juice, salt, and pepper.

5. Pour the filling into the prepared pan (or leave it in the Dutch oven). Spread the mashed sweet potato over the top. Sprinkle with the Pepita Parmesan and rosemary. Bake for about 15 minutes, until the top is crispy and golden. Serve immediately. Leftovers will keep in an airtight container in the fridge for up to 4 days.

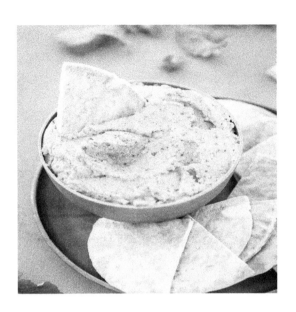

Artichoke-Kale Hummus

SERVES 8 TO 12

PREP TIME: **5 minutes**
ACTIVE TIME: **15 minutes**

3 cups cooked chickpeas (or two 15-ounce cans, rinsed and drained)
¼ cup lemon juice
3 tablespoons tahini (gluten-free if necessary)
3 garlic cloves
1 teaspoon ground cumin
1 teaspoon onion powder
¼ teaspoon cayenne pepper
Salt and black pepper to taste
3 cups packed chopped kale

One 14- to 15-ounce can artichoke hearts, rinsed, drained, and quartered if whole

Bread or crackers (gluten-free if necessary)

1. Combine the chickpeas, lemon juice, tahini, garlic, cumin, onion powder, and cayenne in a food processor and process until smooth. Taste and add salt and pepper as needed. If the dip is too thick, add water by the tablespoon until it reaches your desired thickness.

2. Add the kale and artichoke hearts and pulse until fully incorporated but still chunky. Serve immediately with bread or crackers or refrigerate until ready to use. Leftovers will keep in an airtight container in the fridge for 1 to 2 days.

VARIATIONS

▶ For those who hate hummus (*Who hates hummus?*), switch out the chickpeas with white beans and replace the tahini with olive oil.

▶ For kale haters, switch out the kale for spinach, chard, or collard greens. For those who hate greens altogether, they can be left out completely.

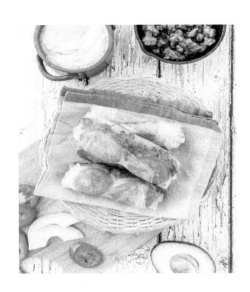

BLT Summer Rolls with Avocado

MAKES 8 ROLLS

PREP TIME: **15 minutes** (not including time to make Quick Bacon Crumbles and Avocado Ranch Dressing or Lemon Dill Aïoli)
ACTIVE TIME: **25 minutes**

Quick Bacon Crumbles (or 10 oz vegan bacon of your choice)
1 small head romaine lettuce, separated into leaves, each leaf chopped in half widthwise
2 to 3 Roma tomatoes, seeded and thinly sliced lengthwise
1 avocado, pitted, peeled, and sliced, optional
Eight 8-inch sheets rice paper (see Tip)
Avocado Ranch Dressing or Lemon Dill Aïoli

1. Fill a large bowl with warm water. Make sure you have a clean surface to prepare the rolls on.

2. Dip a sheet of rice paper into the water, making sure to get it completely wet but removing it quickly before it gets too soft. Lay the paper on the clean surface, then lay a few pieces of lettuce on the center of the paper, going from side to side and leaving about an inch of space around the perimeter. Add a few slices of tomato, a few slices of avocado (if using), and a few spoonfuls of the bacon crumbles (or 2 or 3 slices if you're using a sliced variety).

3. Fold the left and right sides of the paper over the filling. Take the edge of the paper closest to you and fold it completely over the filling while using your fingers to tuck the filling in. Continue rolling until the roll is sealed. Repeat with the remaining ingredients. Serve immediately with the Avocado Ranch Dressing or Lemon Dill Aïoli. These rolls are best enjoyed right after they're made but will keep in an airtight container in the fridge for 5 or 6 hours.

VARIATIONS

For those who aren't fond of avocado, you can leave it out, and switch out the Avocado Ranch Dressing with a regular vegan ranch dressing, or use the Lemon Dill Aïoli.

If your family isn't into summer rolls, just pile all the ingredients between two slices of bread for a sandwich. You won't get any complaints.

TIP

Rice paper sheets that are 6 inches in diameter will be too small.

Perfect Roasted Potatoes

SERVES 4 TO 6

PREP TIME: **10 minutes**
ACTIVE TIME: **10 minutes**
INACTIVE TIME: **40 minutes**

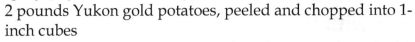

Olive oil spray or vegan cooking spray (soy-free if necessary)

2 pounds Yukon gold potatoes, peeled and chopped into 1-inch cubes

4 tablespoons vegan butter (soy-free if necessary), melted (or ¼ cup olive oil)

2 teaspoons garlic powder

2 teaspoons dried thyme or rosemary

Salt and black pepper to taste

1. Preheat the oven to 400°F . Lightly spray two baking sheets with olive oil.

2. Place the potatoes in a medium pot and cover them with water. Bring to a boil and cook for 5 to 6 minutes, until tender. Drain.

3. Spread out the potatoes on the baking sheets. Use a spatula to gently smash each one just a little bit. Pour the butter over the potatoes. Sprinkle the garlic powder, thyme, salt, and pepper on top. Toss to coat, then spread them out again, making sure that the pieces aren't touching. Bake for 40 minutes, flipping them halfway through. Serve immediately. Leftovers will keep in an airtight container in the fridge for 2 to 3 days.

▶ Feel free to try other seasonings if garlic powder, thyme, or rosemary don't float your boat.

Buffalo Cauliflower Wings with Blue Cheese Dip

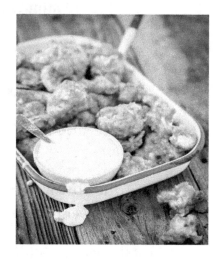

SERVES 4, WITH EXTRA DIP

PREP TIME: **10 minutes**
ACTIVE TIME: **20 minutes** INACTIVE TIME: **15 minutes**

Olive oil spray
buffalo cauliflower
1 cup unsweetened nondairy milk (nut-free if necessary)
1 cup chickpea flour
2 tablespoons cornmeal (gluten-free if necessary)
½ teaspoon garlic powder
½ teaspoon smoked paprika
1 large or 2 small heads cauliflower (2 lb), broken into florets
1 cup hot sauce
2 tablespoons apple cider vinegar
1 tablespoon no-salt-added tomato paste

1 tablespoon maple syrup

blue cheese dip
½ cup plain coconut yogurt (or soy yogurt; unsweetened)
½ cup vegan mayonnaise
2 tablespoons white wine vinegar
½ teaspoon vegan Worcestershire sauce (gluten-free if necessary)
½ teaspoon salt
½ teaspoon garlic powder
¼ teaspoon onion powder
¼ teaspoon dried marjoram
¼ teaspoon dried oregano
Half a 14-ounce block extra firm tofu, drained and crumbled
Black pepper to taste

1. Preheat the oven to 450°F . Lightly spray a 9 × 13-inch baking dish with olive oil.

2. **To make the cauliflower** : Mix the milk, chickpea flour, cornmeal, garlic powder, and paprika in a large bowl. Dredge one cauliflower floret at a time in the mixture and place in the prepared baking dish. Bake for 20 minutes.

3. While the cauliflower is baking, mix together the hot sauce, apple cider vinegar, tomato paste, and maple syrup in a cup or small bowl.

4. Remove the cauliflower from the oven and use a spatula to loosen any florets sticking to the baking dish. Pour the hot sauce mixture over the cauliflower, toss to coat, and bake for 7 to 8 minutes more, until the hot sauce has thickened and caramelized.

5. While the cauliflower is baking the second time, **make the dip** : Mix the yogurt, mayonnaise, white wine vinegar, Worcestershire sauce, salt, garlic powder, onion powder, marjoram, and oregano in a medium bowl. Once combined, fold in the tofu. Taste and add pepper as needed.

6. Serve the cauliflower immediately with the dip. Leftovers will keep in airtight containers in the fridge for 2 to 3 days.

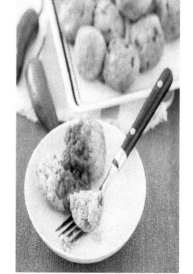

Jalapeño Popper Bites

MAKES 16 TO 18 POPPERS

PREP TIME: **15 minutes** (not including time to cook quinoa)
ACTIVE TIME: **25 minutes**

2 cups cooked quinoa
1 cup <u>corn flour</u> (certified gluten-free if necessary), plus more if needed
3 or 4 small jalapeños, seeded and chopped
2 tablespoons unsweetened nondairy milk (nut-free and/or soy-free if necessary; see Variations)
2 tablespoons lime juice
2 tablespoons vegan cream cheese or mayonnaise (soy-free if necessary)
3 tablespoons nutritional yeast
1 teaspoon ground cumin
½ teaspoon ground coriander

½ teaspoon smoked paprika
Salt and black pepper to taste
Sunflower or canola oil for frying
Salsa

1. Combine the quinoa, corn flour, jalapeños, milk, lime juice, cream cheese or mayonnaise, nutritional yeast, cumin, coriander, and paprika in a large bowl and mix until fully combined. It should be moist and hold together when squeezed, but not wet like batter. If it's too wet, add corn flour by the tablespoon until you have the right consistency. Add salt and pepper.

2. Line a baking sheet with parchment paper or a silicone baking mat. Scoop about 2 tablespoons of the mixture into your hand and shape it into a ball. Place on the prepared baking sheet. Repeat with the remaining mixture.

3. Heat a large frying pan, preferably cast iron, over medium heat. Pour in enough oil to coat the bottom and heat for 2 to 3 minutes. It is important to give the oil enough time to heat. (The bites will fall apart if the oil is not hot enough.) Check to make sure it's hot enough by adding a pinch of the dough to the pan. If it sputters and sizzles, the oil is ready. Line a plate with paper towels.

4. Carefully place 5 or 6 bites in the pan and cook for 3 to 4 minutes, until golden and firm, flipping them every 30 seconds or so to cook on all sides. Use a slotted spoon to transfer them to the plate, placing more paper towels on top to absorb the excess oil. Repeat with the remaining bites, adding more oil to the pan as needed (allow the oil to heat each time you add more). Serve warm, with salsa for dipping. These are best eaten the same day but will keep in an airtight container in the fridge for 1 to 2 days.

VARIATIONS

▶ Make these poppers extra hot by replacing half or all of the milk with hot sauce.

111

To bake the poppers instead of frying them, preheat the oven to 375ºF (190ºC), place the poppers on a baking sheet lined with parchment paper or a silicone baking mat, and bake for 30 minutes, flipping once halfway through.

Cheesy Spiced Popcorn

SERVES 4 TO 6

PREP TIME: **5 minutes**
ACTIVE TIME: **10 minutes**

3 tablespoons nutritional yeast
2 teaspoons chili powder
½ teaspoon garlic powder
A few pinches of cayenne pepper
2 tablespoons sunflower oil (or canola oil)
½ cup popcorn kernels
1 tablespoon vegan butter (soy-free if necessary, or coconut oil), melted
Salt to taste

1. In a small cup or bowl, mix together the nutritional yeast, chili powder, garlic powder, and cayenne pepper. Set aside.

2. Combine the oil and 3 popcorn kernels in a large pot and heat over medium-high heat. Once the kernels pop, add the remaining kernels, cover the pot, shake it a couple of times, and return to the heat. Once the popping begins, continue to shake it every 3 to 5 seconds until the popping stops. Remove from the heat and uncover.

3. Pour the melted butter over the popcorn, cover the pot again, and shake to coat. Uncover the pot and add the nutritional yeast mix, cover again, and shake to coat. Uncover the pot and add salt. Serve immediately.

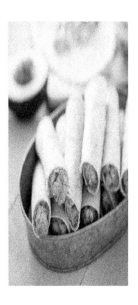

Chickpea-Avocado Taquitos

MAKES 8 TAQUITOS

PREP TIME: **5 minutes**
ACTIVE TIME: **25 minutes**   INACTIVE TIME: **20 minutes**

1½ cups cooked chickpeas (or one 15-ounce can, rinsed and drained)

2 tablespoons liquid aminos (or gluten-free tamari; use coconut aminos to be soy-free)

1 avocado, pitted

2½ tablespoons lime juice

2 green onions, chopped (green and white parts)

1½ tablespoons plain vegan yogurt (or mayonnaise; soy-free if necessary), optional, to add creaminess

½ teaspoon ancho chile powder

½ teaspoon garlic powder

Salt and black pepper to taste

8 corn tortillas (see Tip)

Olive oil spray

Salsa or dip of your choice

1. Preheat the oven to 350°F. Line a baking sheet with parchment paper or a silicone baking mat.

2. Heat a large frying pan, preferably cast iron, over medium heat. Add the chickpeas and liquid aminos and cook, stirring occasionally, until all the liquid has been absorbed. Remove from the heat and let cool for 2 to 3 minutes. Use a potato masher or pastry cutter to mash the chickpeas into small pieces.

3. Scoop the avocado flesh into a large bowl and mash until smooth but slightly chunky. Add the chickpeas, lime juice, green onions, yogurt (if using), ancho chile powder, garlic powder, salt, and pepper. Stir until combined.

4. Heat a frying pan over medium heat and heat the tortillas, one at a time, for 30 seconds on each side, until soft and pliable. Stack them on a plate and cover with aluminum foil while you cook the rest.

5. Lay out 1 tortilla and spread about 3 tablespoons of the avocado mixture down the center. Roll into a tube and place it seam side down on the prepared baking sheet. Repeat with the remaining tortillas and filling.

6. Spray the taquitos with olive oil and bake for 10 minutes. Flip the taquitos, spray them with olive oil again, and bake for another 10 minutes, or until crispy. Serve immediately with your choice of dip or salsa.

VARIATIONS

You can make taquitos with a plethora of different fillings. Try Jackfruit Carnitas, 15-Minute Refried Beans with Pepperjack Cheese Sauce, Tempeh Sloppy Joes, or even Scrambled Tofu .

TIP

Thin corn tortillas work best for these taquitos. Steer away from ones that say "handmade," as those are generally thicker and more likely to crack when you roll them up.

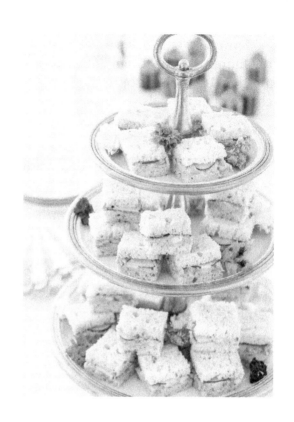

Avocado & Hearts of Palm Tea Sandwiches

MAKES 16 SANDWICHES

PREP TIME: **5 minutes**
ACTIVE TIME: **15 minutes**

2 avocados, pitted
2 teaspoons lemon juice
½ cup finely chopped hearts of palm

Salt and black pepper to taste
8 vegan bread slices (gluten-free if necessary; see Tip)
2 tablespoons chopped fresh parsley
1 cup very thinly sliced radishes

1. Scoop the avocado flesh into a medium bowl and mash until mostly smooth. Add the lemon juice, hearts of palm, salt, and pepper.

2. Spread the avocado mixture on 4 bread slices. Sprinkle with parsley and top with radish slices. Cover each with another piece of bread.

3. Use a bread knife to cut the crusts off each sandwich, then slice each sandwich into four triangles or squares. Serve immediately or refrigerate the sandwiches in an airtight container for up to 3 hours before serving.

TIP

When using gluten-free bread, if you toast it lightly before using, it sometimes tastes better and doesn't dry out as much.

Roasted Red Pepper Hummus Cucumber Cups

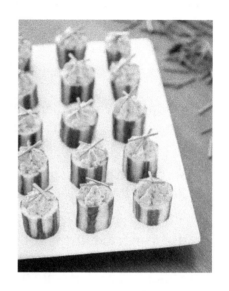

MAKES 30 CUCUMBER CUPS

PREP TIME: **8 minutes**
ACTIVE TIME: **15 minutes**

roasted red pepper hummus
1½ cups cooked chickpeas (or one 15-ounce can, rinsed and drained)
½ cup chopped roasted red peppers
2 garlic cloves
3 tablespoons tahini (gluten-free if necessary)
3 tablespoons lemon juice
½ teaspoon smoked paprika
Pinch of cayenne pepper
Salt and black pepper to taste

cucumber cups
4 English cucumbers
Smoked paprika for dusting
Chives, sliced into 1-inch pieces

1. **To make the hummus** : Combine the ingredients in a food processor and process until smooth, pausing to scrape the sides as necessary. You may need to add water along the way to help smooth it out, but you want a thick hummus. Transfer the hummus to a pastry bag or a large resealable plastic bag with the corner cut out. Chill until ready to use.

2. Trim the ends of the cucumbers. Peel strips of skin from the sides of the cucumbers so you have a striped pattern. Alternatively, you can peel them completely, or not peel them at all. Slice the cucumbers into 1-inch sections. Use a melon baller or a teaspoon to hollow out the insides of the cucumbers, leaving a thick section at one end so that the "cup" has a bottom. Place all of the cups on a plate or platter.

3. Fill each cup with hummus, piling a little on top. Dust the tops with paprika and place 1 or 2 chive pieces on top. Refrigerate until you're ready to serve, up to 1 hour. Leftover hummus will keep refrigerated in an airtight container for 4 to 5 days.

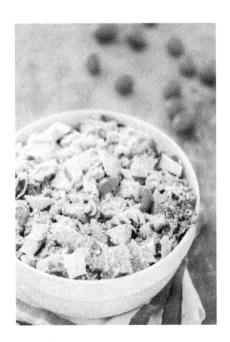

Chickpea Caesar Pasta Salad

SERVES 6 TO 8

PREP TIME: **10 minutes** (not including time to make Pepita Parmesan)
ACTIVE TIME: **30 minutes** INACTIVE TIME: **2 hours**

caesar dressing

¼ cup raw cashews, soaked in warm water for 1 hour and drained, water reserved
6 tablespoons reserved soaking water
¼ cup hemp seeds
3 tablespoons lemon juice
2 tablespoons olive oil
1 tablespoon vegan mayonnaise (soy-free if necessary), optional
1 tablespoon nutritional yeast
2 teaspoons vegan Worcestershire sauce (gluten-free and/or soy-free if necessary)
2 teaspoons Dijon mustard (gluten-free if necessary)
2 teaspoons drained capers
1 garlic clove
Salt and black pepper to taste

salad

12 ounces pasta shape of your choice (gluten-free if necessary)
3 cups cooked chickpeas (or two 15-ounce cans, rinsed and drained)
¼ cup liquid aminos (use coconut aminos to be soy-free)
2 cups halved cherry or grape tomatoes
1 large head romaine lettuce, chopped
2 avocados, pitted, peeled, and chopped
Pepita Parmesan

1. **To make the dressing** : Combine all of the ingredients in a food processor or blender and process until smooth. Set aside.

2. Bring a large pot of water to a boil and cook the pasta according to the package instructions until al dente. Drain, rinse the pasta with cold water, then drain again. Transfer the pasta to a large bowl.

3. Heat a large frying pan, preferably cast iron, over medium heat. Add the chickpeas and liquid aminos and cook, stirring occasionally, until all of the liquid has been absorbed, 4 to 5 minutes. Remove from the heat and add to the pasta.

4. Let the chickpeas cool for 5 to 10 minutes. Add the tomatoes, lettuce, and dressing and toss until combined. Gently fold in the avocado. Cover and refrigerate for 1 hour, or up to 3 hours, before serving. Serve topped with Pepita Parmesan (you can add it to the large bowl if people are serving themselves, or over individual servings if that's how you're serving it). This is best when eaten the day it's prepared but will keep in an airtight container in the fridge for about 1 day.

Sun-Dried Tomato & White Bean Bruschetta

SERVES 10 TO 12

PREP TIME: **10 minutes**
ACTIVE TIME: **15 minutes**

1 long vegan baguette (or other crusty bread; gluten-free if necessary)

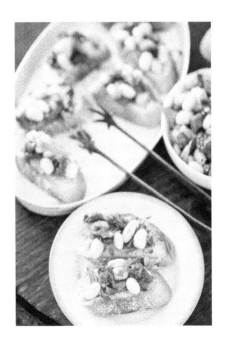

1½ cups cooked cannellini beans (or one 15-ounce can, rinsed and drained)
¾ cups oil-packed sun-dried tomatoes, well drained and diced small
1 garlic clove, crushed
2 tablespoons fresh basil chiffonade
3 tablespoons white wine vinegar
Salt and black pepper to taste
½ cup toasted pine nuts (or other toasted nut or seed), optional
½ cup chopped green onions, optional

1. Preheat the oven to 350°F. Slice the bread into ½-inch slices and arrange them on a baking sheet. Bake for 7 to 10 minutes, until crispy and toasted. Set aside.

2. While the bread is toasting, mix together the beans, tomatoes, garlic, basil, vinegar, salt, and pepper.

3. Scoop some bean mixture onto each of the toasts and sprinkle the tops with pine nuts and green onions (if using). Serve immediately.

TIP

▸ You can prepare the bruschetta topping a few hours in advance and chill until ready to use.

▸ If you have leftover bean mixture, it makes a great filling for a wrap or sandwich.

CPSIA information can be obtained
at www.ICGtesting.com
Printed in the USA
BVHW041409050321
601819BV00007B/259